Slow Train

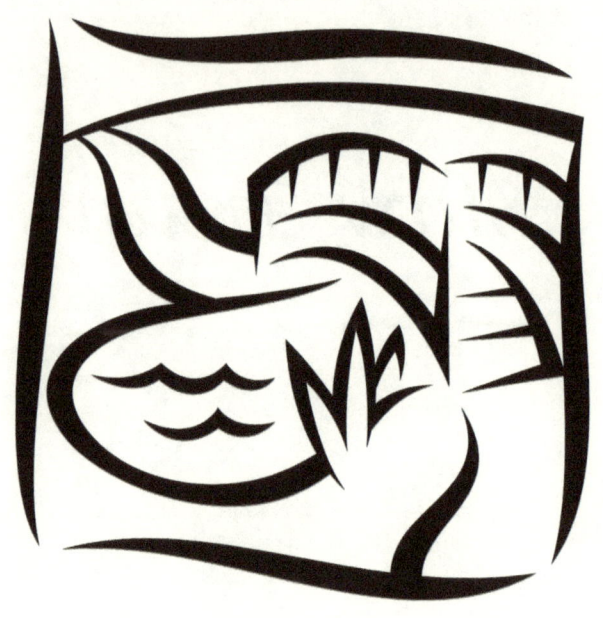

As I stood on the bridge that arched between my old life and my new, so much awareness and understanding flooded in.

Also by Dee Shemma

Climb That Mountain

And coming soon . . .

Companion

Slow Train

A Cancer Journey

DEE SHEMMA

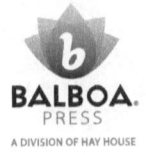

BALBOA.
PRESS

A DIVISION OF HAY HOUSE

Balboa Press books may be ordered through booksellers or by contacting:

Balboa Press
A Division of Hay House
1663 Liberty Drive
Bloomington, IN 47403
www.balboapress.com
1-(877) 407-4847

ISBN: 978-1-4525-4135-8 (sc)
ISBN: 978-1-4525-4136-5 (hc)
ISBN: 978-1-4525-4134-1 (e)

Library of Congress Control Number: 2011914610

Printed in the United States of America

Balboa Press rev. date: 6/11/2012

For my cherished family,
Motti, Aviv and Tali,
With Infinite Love & Gratitude.

AND

To all the beautiful, dear, special,
wounded
Champs who travel the cancer journey,
I wish you
strength, courage and a safe arrival at
your
destination—
perfect, vibrant and lasting health.

"It's only when we truly know and understand that we have a limited time on earth—and that we have no way of knowing when our time is up—that we will begin to live each day to the fullest, as if it was the only one we had."

Elizabeth Kubler-Ross

TABLE OF CONTENTS

Tears **1**

In The Beginning **3**

My Life Before Cancer 5

Diagnosis **6**

On Hearing The Cancer Diagnosis 12

Oh No, I'm Going To **13**

I'm Going To Live Every Day And 14

Self-Help **15**

Candle *21*

'Hair' Today And Gone Tomorrow **22**

Letting Go Of My 'Crowning Glory' 28

Wig On → Wig Off **29**

Love Is . . . When Your Daughter Kisses
Your Bald Head And Tells You That You're
Beautiful! 35

First Chemotherapy **36**

Chemotherapy And Me 46

Side-Effects **47**

Coping With The Side Effects 54

Pain Control **55**

When I'm In Pain 57

Life's Like A Movie **58**

My Life Now 61

Neutropenia **62**

Oyster Shell. *66*

Gran-isms **67**

Help From 'The Other Side' 71

Affirmations **72**

My Own Affirmations 77

Doctors **78**

My Doctors 83

Chemo Pal. **84**

A Special Chemo Friend 88

Mails From The Heart To The Soul **89**

Heart *92*

Genetic Testing **93**

Will I?—Won't I? 98

SCAN SCARED! 99

Surgery **101**

Love Is . . . When Your Teenage Son
Switches Roles With You And He Becomes
The Mum! 109

Liberation Day! **110**

The Day My Life Changed Forever 111

'Sisters'. **112**

My 'Sisters' 115

Where Are You? **116**

I'm Devastated Because 119

Grace **120**

How Grace Touched My Life 122

Gifts **123**

Gifts & What They Meant To Me 125

Contact **126**

The Kind Of Contact I Have/Need 128

50 . . . .**129**

My _____ Cancer Journey Birthday 131

Doctor's Visit's **132**

Doctor's Visits 135

Wellness **136**

My Wellness Programme 141

Depression **142**

When I'm Depressed 147

What Not To Do Or Say! **148**

It Takes All Kinds **154**

Untangling The 'Salad' In My Head 158

A Journey Ends **159**

Losing A Friend To Cancer 165

Read & Know **166**

Spiral *168*

Best Books **169**

Wise & Meaningful Books 172

Carers **173**

Bless Their Beautiful & Unconditionally
Loving Hearts 176

Stuff You Should Know **177**

Not Afraid **180**

My Greatest Fears 183

My Deepest Sadness 184

The Universe **185**

I Ask, Let Go, Trust And Wait 189

Signs And Symptoms **190**

Feather *194*

Prayers, Good Energy & Healing **195**

HELP ME! 197

I Pray 198

Living In The Moment—Now **199**

Letting Go Of The Past & The Future 201

It Ain't Over Till It's Over **202**

How I Feel Now That Treatments Are
Over 205

Send It Back **206**

I'm Finished With Cancer Forever 208

The Gift Of Cancer **209**

Cancer Brought Me Many Gifts 212

Benefits 213

Benefits Available To Me 216

Cancer Profile 217

My Profile, As I See Myself Now 219

Things To Get Used To 220

Getting Used To _____ Was Hard
For Me 223

First Hair Cut 224

The Joy Of Having Hair Again 227

Recovery 228

My Recovery 234

6 Months Down The Road 235

6 Months Later 241

The One Year Milestone 242

12 Months Later 247

Flower 248

Gym Judgement 249

My New Exercise Plan 252

Lessons Learned 253

LOVE THE LESSON! 260

I Learned That 261

And Another Thing 262

OVERCOME! 264

Acorn 265

Long-Term Survivial **266**

I'm A Survivor. I'm A Long-Term
Survivor 271

Help From 'The Others'! **272**

How I Can Make A Difference Now 277

Born Again **278**

My New Life 283

The End **285**

Who Am I? **287**

Poems-Prayers-Pieces **289**

SCAN SCARED! 289

OVERCOME!. 291

HELP ME! 292

LOVE THE LESSON! 293

Affirmations **294**

The 'Famous Folder' **296**

Chemotherapy Checklist. **299**

THIS BOOK

Preface

Slow Train comes to you from the still place between two heart beats, where all our answers lie. I've written from the chambers of my heart and the deepest layers of my soul.

You may wonder at the appropriateness of the title *Slow Train*. I'll tell you how it came about. One day, shortly after the cancer diagnosis, I was out driving. My mind was in a whirlwind and I was trying desperately to nail my mind down to focus on the task in hand, just driving. My whole being felt hollow due to the sheer weight and magnitude of what lay ahead for me. You could have crushed me with a feather. When I finally got my mind back on one track, I became aware of Katie Melua's velvety voice crooning on the CD player—"I'm just a slow train crawling up a hill." Rewind, listen, again, rewind and listen, again, again and again, until the words seeped in through my skin. Oh, how right they felt, that was **exactly** how I felt. And so it was!

Trains are strong. Even if they climb a hill slowly, they get there in the end, pulling any size load. You can be a slow train, climbing and crawling up a hill—it may take time, but you **will** get there in the end.

The word 'Champ' in *Slow Train* is short for the word 'champion'—my understanding of, and name for, the woman doing the cancer journey.

Please note that throughout *Slow Train* I use the word God, Universe or otherwise interchangeably—please read the word to mean "The God of <u>your</u> understanding."

In *Slow Train*, 'he' refers to the doctor and 'she' the Champ.

I don't talk about 'my' cancer, say "I have cancer" or 'own' it in any way—just 'the' cancer.

You will note that there is little mention of radiotherapy or radiation treatments in *Slow Train*. I barely referred to them because I didn't do those treatments myself and decided not to write about treatments I know very little about.

During the journey, I don't think I managed to read any book from beginning to end. I didn't have either the focus or the energy. I dipped into books, I browsed, I paged through and I looked at books. *Slow Train* is written with complete understanding and empathy of how your journey really is, dear Champs. So:

o Each chapter is complete in itself, so you can dip into *Slow Train* and read any chapter at random.
o The type is large and clear, knowing that you may have blurred vision during chemo.
o The book itself is a size that could fit in your handbag, be held comfortably when

lying down or sitting in a queue waiting for a doctor's consultation, test or scan.

o The ten images are for days when you don't have energy to even read; you can just look at the images and absorb the wisdom of the captions, possibly prompting a meditation or moments of mindfulness.

o After most of the chapters there is a page where you can journal your own feelings, thoughts, or notes on what you have read.

o The Table of Contents lists the Chapters, Images, Poems-Prayers-Pieces and the Journal Pages in different fonts, so that you can access what you are looking for at a glance.

o The chapters are short, knowing that you may be too tired, unwell or unable to concentrate for long periods of time.

o The four Poems-Prayers-Pieces throughout the book may also be found, together, on pages 208-211, for easy access at a later date, if you should need them.

o You'll find all the affirmations mentioned in *Slow Train* grouped on page 212.

o Tips on how to manage your 'Famous Folder' can be found on pages 213-214.

o When in a hurry to pack for a day at the Chemo Unit just check out pages 215-216, where you will find a Chemotherapy Checklist.

- Most of all, *Slow Train* is infused with great love, light, compassion and fervent wishes for your journey and arrival at a healthy, happy and healed place.

I have five goals in writing this book:

- I want to share my story.
- It's my dearest wish that *Slow Train* will be a comforting companion (giving validation) to fellow Champs as they journey to perfect, vibrant and lasting health.
- It is my hope that through *Slow Train* readers, who accompany Champs on their journeys, will be able to see into the minds and feel into the hearts and souls of the Champs.
- On the journey I came across so many cancer books that described cancer symptoms, chemotherapy, radiation, pain, diet, what to do and what not to do. I promised myself that once I'd healed, recovered and regained my energy that I'd write about how I felt, how the journey changed me, how I learned, healed and grew.
- Lastly, I want people to see the cancer journey differently, from the side of light, hope and, in time, gratitude.

In the movie 'Australia' the wise old Aborigine says that all you need is love in your heart and your story. My heart is now overflowing with love for all the beautiful souls in my life and I have the story of the journey to share. May the light of *Slow Train* bring you comfort and serenity. **Enjoy!**

ACKNOWLEDGMENTS

With infinite love and gratitude I thank my family for their never-ending belief in me, undying support and unconditional love, no matter what.

I'm enormously grateful to my parents for their love, devotion to duty and all the valuable lessons they taught me that prepared me so well for my life as it is today.

To my Support Circle, whom I don't need to mention by name, because I regularly tell each and every one of you how blessed and grateful I am for the heart and soul connection we enjoy, how truly fortunate I am to have such treasured people in my life and how much I love you all.

Dear readers, you were in my thoughts as the words of *Slow Train* spilled from my heart for you. My foremost wish being to make a difference to even one of your lives, even for a day. I thank you and wish you healing, love and peace.

A special thanks to all the team at Balboa Press, who patiently and efficiently walked with me through every step of the publishing process.

TEARS

Tears will come even if you are not generally a tearful or emotional person. You won't plan it. They may come when you least expect it, but they will come, lots of them and possibly often.

I cried just looking at my food and not having the energy to lift my fork.

I cried when walking the eight paces, from the kitchen to my recycling bin, seemed overwhelming.

I cried when I 'crashed' every time I came off steroids.

I cried when at 9.30 a.m. (that's morning!) I knew my day was over (energy-wise) and yet it hadn't even begun.

I cried in the shower, my tears falling in harmony with the water, just because I'd made it to the end of another day.

I cried when everything seemed too much for me to handle.

I cried when I looked in the mirror and didn't recognize myself.

I cried when I watched my daughter coming out of school chatting to friends. I cried tears of begging that I would be around to share more of her growing up, be the one to hold her hand and mother her into adulthood.

I cried when my wig felt hot and tight.

I cried when, even with pain relief, I couldn't handle the pain.

I cried when the journey seemed endless at times.

I cried with joy when people 'got it' and knew how to handle me and help me in the way I needed.

I cried from relief when I fell into bed.

I cried when I missed sharing important events in my son's life.

I cried when my life felt like the life of a very old person.

I cried when I tried to keep up and failed miserably.

I cried silently in my heart many times and no tears fell at all.

I cried when my blood test results didn't portray my mammoth effort at wellness.

I cried when getting a simple meal on the table for my family felt like running two marathons.

A lot of the time I had no idea why I was crying, I just was.

Tears came. They didn't always last long but I let them come for as long as they needed to. It brought me relief just to let go. It felt human. I knew that when I cried I was in my heart, as opposed to my head and this was the perfect place to start healing.

IN THE BEGINNING

"To heck with this 'fifty' thing, I'm just not doing it," I declared, as I tried to hike myself up on the freezer, in order to lean down and retrieve the hose of the hoover that had just fallen behind it. But, not today it seemed. I just couldn't seem to lift myself up. I was in complete and utter disbelief. I was after all, only forty-nine years old (generally feeling about twenty-nine), physically fit and usually brim full of energy. This was the first sign, for me, that something was amiss. It was August 2008.

Within a week I needed a daily nap. Weeks later I was going to bed early and napping four times a day. Everyday life became a struggle, I lost my healthy appetite and people began to comment on my pale face, dramatic weight loss and lack of zest for life.

My spirit felt drained, my body was on strike and every part of me was screaming "No more." My soul wasn't singing and hadn't been singing for a long time, which most likely meant it was either crying or dying. I didn't need a doctor to tell me I was sick, I only needed him to confirm what I already knew—things were not good.

I had many emotions that were very definitely not in motion. The emotions and pain that I'd buried for years were now festering—the seeds of ovarian cancer had been sown.

Pre-cancer I led what I had considered to be a healthy life-style. I exercised, I had an excellent water filter in my kitchen, I ate organic food, my diet was mostly vegetarian, I had never smoked or done drugs, I consumed alcohol sparingly, I meditated, I used alternative cures when I was unwell, I went for regular medical check-ups, visits to the gynecologist and did mammograms. I did all of the above and more. I truly believed that I was taking good care of my health and my body. I could be forgiven for being smug enough to assume that I'd never get cancer, right? I thought cancer was something that happened to people who didn't take care of themselves—other people of course! But here is the big lesson—there is no guarantee with cancer, we are not the ones in charge or control.

On September 4th 2008, I went for my third vaginal ultrasound to monitor a cyst on my right ovary. It had previously been monitored in March and May. As soon as the radiographer completed the scan she looked at me and said "Things are messed up." She sent me, urgently, to my gynecologist.

By the time I arrived at my gynecologist's office, an hour later, the radiographer had already faxed over my report. I could tell that my gynecologist was uncomfortable. She prepared all the relevant referrals for the further testing I'd need to have done, directed me to the hospital where the biopsy would be performed and got me out of her office in a rather hurried manner. I already knew, in my heart, that it was cancer.

MY LIFE BEFORE CANCER . . .

DIAGNOSIS

I clearly remember the sensations in my body on hearing the ovarian cancer diagnosis, over the phone, but it's hard to describe the impact in words—it was, perhaps, akin to watching the Twin Towers collapse. My life as I'd known it to that date (October 23rd 2008) smashed instantly in pieces around me and was over. Assuming that there would be a life post cancer, I knew with great certainty that things would never be the same again, for me! My heart raced, my knees shook, I felt like my soul might have left my body and I couldn't trust my voice box to produce sounds had I chosen to speak. I wasn't focused enough to realize that a different life didn't necessarily mean a worse life, things could also change for the better—which is exactly what happened. Every end, after all, also marks a new beginning.

The diagnosis itself wasn't what shocked me to my core. I already knew that I was very sick and was going downhill fast. I'd been completely and totally wiped out with exhaustion in September. I recall the sheer struggle of getting a meal on the table and performing basic tasks like laundry, driving or emptying the dishwasher. It was all overwhelming and much more than I was able for. I was usually hyper energetic and now I was napping four times a day. As the days progressed it grew harder and more challenging to cope. When I met people while out, I noticed the shocked look on their faces when they saw me. Their eyes dilated and I detected an instant when they wondered whether they should comment on my pale face, my dramatic weight loss and my sick look or just let it pass.

In fact, had the surgeon told me it wasn't cancer I'd have been even more surprised. What rocked me was the enormity of what lay ahead, the unknown, the challenge of survival and the worry that I may not be strong enough to deal with everything that would be thrown in my path over the next year.

I immediately started getting in touch with loved ones. I felt an overwhelming need to share the news and gather as much love, comfort and strength around me as possible. Some instinct, which I heeded, held me back from sharing the news with anyone who I felt might, on hearing the diagnosis, assume I wouldn't make it. I waited till I was comfortable with my new status before venturing into such negative territory.

Everyone I shared my news with reacted with such love and compassion. In fact, they all handled the situation so well that I wondered, if heaven forbid, the tables had been turned, whether I'd have been able to do the same for them with such perfect ease.

I spent the next hour alone, with my thoughts. Never before was my life so crystal clear to me. It was as if the blind-fold had been removed from my eyes, as if the black-out blinds had been pulled open and the fog that had previously clouded my brain's understanding of my life had been lifted. I could see the mistakes I'd made, the time I'd wasted, the things in my life that didn't resonate with my soul, I understood what changes I needed to make and it was clear what I no longer wanted to do with my life. The knowledge of what I really did want to do with my time and my life, from now on, screamed it's message so loud that I heard at last. I was grateful for the first gift of this cancer journey—clarity of mind, heart and soul. I knew what I wanted and, also, what I no longer wanted in my life.

There were two questions to ask myself once I was over the initial impact of shock:

1) Do I want to go on, or not?
2) Am I willing to make the effort it will take to survive?

Once I'd answered 'yes' to both questions I knew I was already at the starting point of my journey. That was all I needed for now. I had a direction. Great!

Following the hour I took to centre and ground myself, I now faced the task of sharing the news with my children. I wanted to be able to tell them without breaking down myself. I knew that I couldn't show any fear, that they would be scared enough, without it appearing that I couldn't cope either. I knew that even though I'd just received an ovarian cancer diagnosis that I was still a mother. How I handled this situation would most likely be how my children would handle it too.

My son was eighteen. My daughter had just turned twelve. I wanted to share the news with them myself. I decided to tell each one separately and privately, thus giving them the space to react naturally, ask questions and take as much time as was necessary for them to absorb how their lives, as well as mine, were in for a marathon roller-coaster ride.

They already knew that the cyst on my right ovary had been monitored in March, May and September. They were on board about the biopsy that had been performed on October 6th. There had never been any secrets that now needed to be uncovered. I spoke slowly, calmly and honestly. I told them the facts and details as I knew them to be. I shared my optimism about whatever treatment would be planned for me and I assured them that I intended to do my utmost to make a full recovery.

Their separate reactions to my news remain private but to this day are engraved in my memory and warm my heart. It was abundantly clear that they were mature, supportive, optimistic and very understandably, a little anxious. They immediately gripped the gravity of the situation but their level of belief in me was more than enough to, later, keep me trying, even on days when I wondered whether the chemo itself might finish me off. I knew my staunchest supporters lived right at home with me. Their unconditional love kept me going during many a dark hour. I looked at each of them and knew that I would use every last ounce of strength in my being to survive this lesson, in order to continue my treasured role as their very fortunate mother.

My son was eighteen and I felt so much gratitude that I'd had the opportunity to raise him to adulthood. I cried, till I felt my heart would split when I contemplated my twelve year old daughter. I just had to survive to raise her myself. I begged to be given the opportunity to also bring her to eighteen . . . and on further contemplation, changed my request to 'whenever', at least!

The gynecology surgeon who'd performed the biopsy would now pass my file on to a gyne/oncologist. Even hearing the word 'oncologist', or saying it, was heavy, shocking and took getting used to.

I had no idea yet what the treatment protocol would be—whether it would involve surgery, chemotherapy, radiation or all three. Time would reveal all and I'd have to be patient and wait—lesson number two, I guess!

I'm not sure whether it was the knowledge of what I already knew, or the fear of what I, as yet, didn't know, that affected my sleep, but my sleep pattern was seriously disrupted and disturbed. It took forever to fall asleep. When I eventually slept it was fitful, anxious and riddled with panic dreams. I woke constantly and my imagination went into unbridled overdrive.

I was afraid. I wasn't afraid of anything specific. It was more like a global fear of the unknown but it was naked, raw and deep-seated. The road ahead just seemed to stretch out before me to infinity and beyond.

It became clear, very quickly, that I'd been harbouring deeply buried emotions that had been screaming for my attention for the longest time. These neglected emotions were still there and were now surfacing at an alarming rate. Had I really imagined that I had all the time in the world to make changes that I had known all along required action? Apparently yes!

What brought the first welcome ray of calm was the realization that I couldn't change the diagnosis but there was a lot I could do to impact the prognosis. If I took responsibility for my situation, it could make all the difference. I thought about how I could work on my own healing, starting with my emotions—right now.

ON HEARING THE CANCER DIAGNOSIS . . .

OH NO, I'M GOING TO . . .

You have just heard your cancer diagnosis. One of the first thoughts that may enter your head is "Oh no, I'm going to die." Well, yes you are, but then, so is everyone else on the planet! It is everyone's destiny to die, not just yours. You may have been diagnosed with cancer but that doesn't mean you are necessarily going to die now—**any** of us can die at **any** time.

What you really need to focus on is not **when** you will die but, rather, **how** you will live **until** you die. There will be people who will look at you, as if you already have 'one foot in your grave', when you tell them you have ovarian cancer, but the point they are missing is that they could be gone before you! There are no age advantages or rules regarding who will die first.

The bottom line is that no one knows when he is going to die (and thank heavens for that!). We are not in charge or control, we are not the ones to decide (and neither is your doctor by the way!) when our lives will end. Our lives will end when they end and, until that moment comes, we have the busy task of living life to the full to get on with.

I'M GOING TO LIVE EVERY DAY AND . . .

SELF-HELP

You won't have to worry about where to start the cancer journey, because once you are diagnosed, you are already on the journey, whether you choose it or not. It's the most effective wake-up call you may ever have!

Most likely you have behaved your way into the life you now live, so it stands to reason then, that you are going to have to behave your way out of it! In real terms, that means making lots of changes.

You may want to scream at the universe, your partner or yourself "Why me?" I'd advise you to take a short cut, bypass that wasteful question, for which there is no answer, or guilty party. Ask, instead, "What am I going to do about this?" This is not a blame game. This is a journey, as you will see in time.

For as long as I can remember I've heard people talking about *fighting* cancer, *waging war* on cancer, *battling* or *tackling* the disease, *defeating* the big 'C' and *beating* 'it'. These words are so hard, so negative, they are words of loss (in violent situations everyone is a loser) and of huge energy expenditure. I think that it's easier to manage by deleting these words of negativity and replacing them with positive, uplifting and softer language, like *letting go*, *healing* and *learning lessons*.

You may have to take time to think about this, but it's my own experience, that when faced with almost every challenging situation I've had to deal with in life, in hindsight, I've noticed that I'd already met such an experience, before I had to experience it personally. Ask any mother who has miscarried and she'll have known another mother who has miscarried before she herself did. When someone's partner ends his/her own life, the surviving partner will have known someone who was in the same position before the experience came into his/her own space. Likewise, when life hands you cancer, you'll already have had some contact beforehand with someone who has already done the journey before you. Unaware, the Universe prepares us before each experience.

In my own case, I was given most of the tools I needed to successfully complete my journey, long before it started. I'd done many healing courses and workshops, I'd read scores of mind/body/spirit books, I have several close friends who are healers, I knew how to meditate, I was aerobically fit, I was already eating organic food, had installed a good water filter in my kitchen, had changed all my body care products to safer ones, had been keen on journaling and more. You might wonder if there was anything else left to do, change or learn—you can't even begin to imagine how much baggage there was to offload and how much learning was required, but, I had my 'tool kit' and I was, thankfully, pretty well prepared.

You may have been a 'type A' personality all your life, organized, liking it when a plan comes together, punctual, prepared and in control—and then you met cancer! The biggest lesson of all with cancer is that we are not the ones in charge or control. Whether it's our nature or not, whether it suits us or not, whether we want to or not, we just have to (sooner or later) learn to wait, let go and flow. It's good for you to understand this before setting off on your journey!

Cancer is a journey, it's a process. Simply put, that means there is no quick fix. Like all good processes, it takes time. The journey is completed a day at a time, a step at a time and a moment at a time. Like all interesting journeys there are corners, hills, bumps, twists and turns on the way and we rarely see the end from where we set off.

It's more important than you can imagine not to 'own' cancer. You might well ask, "How do you do that?" What does that really mean? This very significant strategy I learned from Darren Weissman's book 'The Power of Infinite Love and Gratitude'. He explains that we should not say "My cancer" or "I have cancer."

Everyone who understands about healing will tell you that cancer is about anger. Of course we all negate this when we first hear the news that cancer has paid us a visit. We try to explain how we are not angry but sad, depressed, stressed, tired or in need of a change. In time, the anger will surface and you'll recognize it as anger, not something else (even by name!) when it does. As you journey, you'll let go of anger and replace it with love.

Naturally you will feel fear often and possibly for extended periods of time. Sometimes it can be raw, naked fear and at other times it may be disguised by a different emotion. There are so many potential fear suspects—needles, bad test results, surgery, side-effects of chemo, constant exhaustion, not being able to be part of life, pain and the list is endless. Each Champ has her own most fearful thought, moment or situation.

I would be the last person on the planet to tell you not to feel fear. Was I afraid as I journeyed? Of course I was, often. It bordered on terror at times. I'd say, feel the fear and then let it go. Don't try to pretend you are not afraid or squash it down . . . you won't be able anyhow, no matter how hard you try! Or, as Susan Jeffers so brilliantly advises "Feel the fear and do it anyway."

The thought of death crops up once cancer is mentioned. Personally I don't fear death but I understand why a person might. For me, the idea of not living is much more fearful than death. We will all die at some time or other but will we all be able to say that we have lived? Let this be food for thought for you today. Change your emphasis if you can, it will make the world of difference to you as you plod through this long, tiring and challenging journey.

During the cancer journey my family was incredibly loving and supportive. We spoke about every element of the journey all the time, any time and any place. Now I see things differently. I feel that there should be at least one room, one place, one time, one situation or one day a week when cancer is never discussed. It could be that it's never mentioned at the dining table, or in the children's bedrooms, or till after breakfast or never on Sundays. You can decide. I think our families are so wonderful at this time, but how much can good people be expected to take, without having a break? They need a break from it from time to time and so do you.

One day at the chemo unit I saw a beautifully groomed woman flicking through her diary to see which date would suit her to start her chemotherapy. Not this date, not till after that event and not before the other occasion. That is how one may behave for a very brief time in the beginning, until it becomes abundantly clear that chemotherapy does not fit neatly into your schedule, but the other way around, your life fits around chemotherapy.

There are obvious things like unhealthy food, alcohol, cigarettes and such like to avoid when you are ill. It's clear too that stressful situations and people should not be part of your life at this time. Anything that doesn't resonate with you or irritates your emotions should be cast aside. Just decide you are not doing these things anymore. Period.

19

Take responsibility—you are the one who is sick, so, you are the one who has to work hard to get well again. You are the one who has to make changes and learn lessons, not someone else. Doctors and healers will guide and advise you but you'll be the one doing the work.

Get in touch with your inner thoughts. Connect with your feelings. Sharpen the awareness of the sensations in your body. When you are tuned in to yourself on all levels you will know what you need, what you want and your body will reap the rewards.

It's very important to stay out of sick mode and out of bed whenever you can. Of course the illness is serious, life-threatening, major and beyond hellishly challenging, but if you can be well when you are and get out of bed when you feel you are able to, it will help you to feel that you are part of 'the land of the living' and that you have a life, a different life, but none-the-less, a life.

If you have been a busy, busy, busy person all your life, as I had been, then it's time to sit down and think of all the ways in which you can (and will) slow your life down. At first you think you can't cut anything out, can't let go of so many activities, find it hard to delegate, wonder how things will get done if you are not at the helm, but fear not, life really does carry on beautifully and smoothly even without our input.

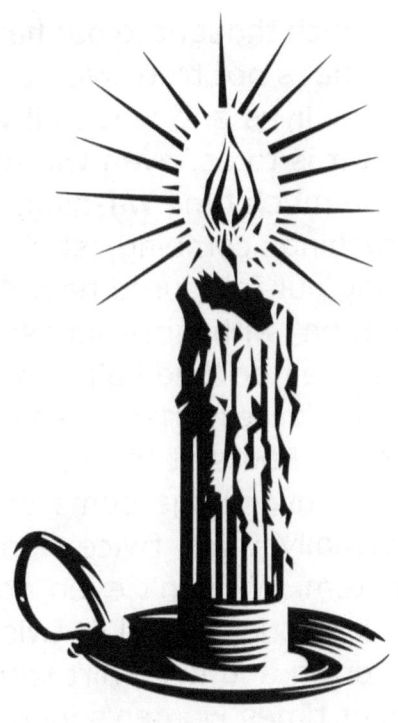

A white light in the darkness will
cleanse your mind & spirit, and heal
emotions that are in turmoil.

'HAIR' TODAY AND
GONE TOMORROW

We don't give much thought to our hair till we don't have any. No, that's not true! We do. Our hair is a huge part of our lives and we're all well aware of how important it is to us, even without losing it.

We spend so much time washing, conditioning, colouring, brushing, combing, styling, arranging and blow-drying our treasured hair. We talk about our hair 'situation' with girl-friends; we bemoan the state of our hair on 'bad hair' days; we pick up hair products and accessories when out shopping; we spend endless hours at the hairdressing salon and gladly hand over huge sums of money that we would normally think twice about spending on any other item. We don't even notice how we constantly fix it, settle it, twirl it, twist it, tie it up, let it cascade down and even flirt with it.

From ancient times women's long, silky, shiny, lush hair has been their pride and joy, their crowning glory. Our hair is a major part of our womanhood, of being feminine and who we are. The style, colour, length and amount of time we devote to it all speak volumes about us.

In light of all this, try then to imagine how it would feel to lose your hair. Losing all her hair is a major life event for any woman—even for the woman who says she doesn't mind!

Losing your hair early on the chemotherapy journey is yet another ordeal for you to deal with and a rather high hill to climb. You have already, in quick succession, learned that you are no longer healthy, that you have cancer, you are going to have possible multiple surgeries, radiation, chemotherapy and a long crawl back to the recovery of your health; you have been informed of a whole menu of side-effects that will wreak havoc on your wellbeing and daily life; you have been told that this journey is not a sprint but a marathon; no one needed to mention it at all but it is abundantly clear that many Champs, in your situation, don't make it. Now, on top of all that, with as much dignity as you can muster, you try to grapple with the impending loss of your hair.

There was a deadline in sight. I'd been informed at the chemo unit, that my hair would start to fall out, around ten days after I received the first round of chemotherapy. At first I said I'd just wait and let it all fall out naturally—not a very bright choice, in hindsight!

Shortly afterwards I was fortunate enough to cross paths with a cancer survivor who had also done chemo. A brief chat with her put me straight. During chemo, hair doesn't fall out one hair at a time but in large clumps, randomly, over your head. It was clear that I didn't want clumps of hair falling out all over the house. It would be akin to having the largest, hairiest dog you can imagine molting in my house. You can now multiply that by ten of course for speed of loss and amount of hair **everywhere**. Everywhere includes, on you, anyone you hug, your bed, floor, couch and possibly in your food! The visual, for me, of how it would be for my children, to sit with me at dinner, with clumps of hair missing all over my head was enough for me to speed-decide to have my head shaved.

I had no regrets whatsoever about doing this. In the end it was easier for me and, without a shadow of a doubt, it was less traumatic for my family.

Look at it this way, anyway within days all my hair would have fallen out by itself. By shaving my head a few days earlier I ended up with the same result, but minus the trauma.

Needless to add, I shed tears—the quiet silent type, about my hair loss. It wasn't that I'd loved my hair (the colour or even the style), it was about this being another hurdle for me to overcome, hopefully without falling flat on my face. I had yet another thing to let go of—yet another new angle to my, by now, upside-down life.

But, like everything else in life, we have a huge capacity for dealing with change and we are capable of far more than we realize.

I was doing quite well with the prospect of having my head shaved . . . until the morning the appointment swung around. I was shaking inside, my heart felt like lead and my knees were not to be trusted. I saw my daughter off to school and crawled back into the safety of my bed and the cozy comfort of my quilt to hide. I put on a meditation CD, closed my eyes and felt my feelings—all of them.

As I closed my eyes, tears trickled down my cheeks on the, by now, familiar route to my chin. Then, without any planning, something magical happened. I saw a vision of myself as a toddling two year old, with my blond wavy hair like a halo around my face. She smiled and floated away. In her place I recognized a familiar seven-year-old. There I stood in all my glory, with my now darker, straight hair, my neat, short style. She ran off to play. I found myself looking at a head of thick, waist-length, auburn hair. This twelve-year-old smiled and vanished. Next I was a student, peddling along on my bicycle to college, with the wind sweeping through my newly permed hair. I felt light and free.

As the music warmed and comforted the tears in my heart and the vibrations of my soul, the images floated towards me and vanished, as I visually worked my way through the various hair 'stages' of my life. The final 'me' gave a reassuring smile and a nod before departing.

Gratitude flooded through me. The angels were helping me to let go of my hair in the gentlest way possible. They were helping me to see the beauty of my hair at all the stages of my life, right from when I was a little girl to date and to be grateful for what I'd had. On seeing the frames of each stage I have to admit to feeling such warmth and love for those times and memories, which had long since been forgotten.

I was ready now, quietly strong and just a tiny bit shaky inside, if I'm being totally honest. Mostly I felt calm and in full acceptance of what lay ahead. It was the right thing for me to do, for now. I know those around me worried that I might crack so I decided to avoid all eye contact and stay in my own, now protected, space.

The staff at the wig shop could not have been more sympathetic, (without being mushy), kind, understanding and pleasant. They were well-experienced in handling situations such as mine. Without further delay (they knew not to prolong the agony of the final moments), I was brought downstairs to a small booth, with a mirror (I thought that was interesting!) and the most compassionate hairdresser. Till today I can recall her face, her empathy and connection to my plight.

She asked if I wanted to turn my chair away from the mirror. No, I felt I could handle watching. As the first band of hair was whisked away, my eyes welled with tears but no tear fell. I was okay. My whole head was shaved at the speed of light, in what seemed like seconds.

And wow, here I saw another gift—my new look was cute! I actually preferred my shaved look to the 'me' with a full head of hair. For the first time ever I noticed the shape of my head and fell in love with it instantly! My eyes looked huge and really were a feature now. When had I ever paid attention to my lips at all? Well, I could really see them now. I exhaled a gigantic sigh of relief—it was done. It was another step forward. I'd managed better than I'd anticipated.

As soon as my head was shaved the kind hairdresser offered me a wig to wear while my own was being adjusted to the smaller, shrunken size of my newly shaved head. I didn't need it. I was fine about being bald. It wasn't anywhere nearly as terrible as I'd originally imagined it might have been.

LETTING GO OF MY 'CROWNING GLORY' . . .

WIG ON → WIG OFF

The choice to wear a wig or not is entirely personal. Some women choose to wear bandanas all the time, while others decide that they feel more comfortable going around bald. Having done the journey, I felt I looked more 'normal' either bald or with a wig. The bandana look seemed to draw more attention. I felt I looked really ill when I wore a bandana.

Some days you feel like going around bald. Other days you feel that a cotton bandana is more comfortable and fits your mood (or even the weather) that day. Yet there are days, times, places and situations when you may feel like blending in and being less noticeable; you may feel like looking more 'normal'; you may not feel up to answering all the questions, or deal with knowing stares, that may accompany the 'bald' or 'bandana' look; there will be days when you feel well and want to dress up a bit, go out and look good. For whatever reason, it's very nice to have a wig on hand for the days when you don't feel like wearing a bandana, being bald and you want to look more like 'the old' you. Having one at home gives you a choice.

I, for example, always wore my wig to my daughter's school (even when I didn't get out of the car). I always wore it to functions, my local mall and to restaurants. When I was at home alone I choose to wear neither bandana nor wig. At all other times I wore bandanas—for walks on the beach, meeting close friends, going for alternative treatments, on days at the chemo unit and when I was out for breakfast with friends and the wig became too hot, tight or was irritating my head, I'd go to the bathroom and change into my bandana. Wig on, wig off, just became second nature to me and a way of life that no longer cost me a thought. Proof yet again that us humans really can get used to just about anything.

Having been informed that my hair would start to fall out about ten days after receiving the first chemo treatment, I knew I'd have to make a move on getting a wig. I made an appointment for the morning after I'd received my first treatment. In hindsight, this was a huge mistake. You might ask, "Why?"

Well, the day of the first chemo was so long and I'd been quite anxious in the preceding days, that I was now understandably exhausted. I hadn't factored in that I might already feel unwell. As it turned out I woke up, that morning, with an allergy to the one of the chemo drugs. My neck and face were roaring red. I couldn't wear any make-up. I looked hellish from the drugs and the 'experience' of the previous day. I was weary, stunned and out of focus. It was the wrong day to sit under the bright lights of a hairdresser/wig shop mirror and make an important decision regarding the wig that I'd be wearing for the coming year. I wasn't capable of making the correct choices that day . . .

but I did, because I was there and wasn't sure whether I'd feel any better, stronger or more like doing this tomorrow than I did today.

I still had all my own hair and was fitting wigs on over it. My heart wasn't in it at all and yet I tried to grip the importance of it. At one point I looked in the mirror but didn't see myself at all. What came into view and clear focus was the row of chairs behind me. There I saw women sitting waiting, after head-shaving and women who were already bald and having their wigs adjusted, washed or styled. I was completely transported away from my own reality. Tears stung my eyes and my heart welled with empathy and pity. I scanned these dignified women with my emotions as opposed to my eyes. Wow, the word "Braveheart" took on a whole new meaning for me that day. Each woman with her own story, pain, fears, issues to deal with, lessons to learn and her own exhaustion. Each woman staying as calm and quiet as she could—so that she herself could cope better by zoning out and possibly in an effort to make it easier for the women sitting on either side of her.

I heard my name being called and I blinked my eyes tightly a couple of times to bring myself back to the reality of my wig choice.

A wig needs to be chosen as carefully as possible and there are a few reasons for this, mostly the cost. Wigs are frightfully expensive, even the cheap ones! It's unlikely that you will buy more than one wig for the duration of the chemo journey. You will want to get it as right as you can because you will be the one wearing it, possibly day in and day out, for the bones of the next year!

Buy the most expensive wig you can afford—it will be your 'hair' for so long and you want to look as well as you can, even if you are sick.

Choosing the style is the 'fun' bit here. If you love your hair-style as it is then you may go for a similar style. If you are the type of person who doesn't want people to 'notice' that your wig is a wig, then, also, go for a style as close as you can to your own. If you've always dreamed of having long, wavy, shoulder-length hair then go for it, now is a golden opportunity to check it out. How you choose it is entirely up to you. Remember a wig is not something you can buy on a whim and change your mind about later.

In my own case, I chose a wig that was very close to the colour and texture of my own natural hair. In fact, the quality of the wig hair was superior to my own. The style wasn't what I wanted but that didn't matter. I learned that a wig can be styled, permed, coloured, cut and highlighted, just the same as real hair can. So, getting the quality and texture right is the best start, after that you can 'play around' with the 'effects'.

Fortunately for me I was too tired to make any decisions on my own that day, so, I listened and 'obeyed' the hairdresser. She was very experienced and knew her trade well. She advised me to just have a slight trim that day, wear the wig for a week to see how it felt and only then come back for the 'real' cut. She wisely pointed out the obvious, that once it's cut, it won't grow again like your own hair and a mistake is a mistake you will be stuck with for a long time.

Sitting at the side while adjustments were made to my wig, I found myself unable to concentrate enough to read. My eyes fell on a young woman, about twenty-seven years old. She was sobbing very quietly to herself. I so understood the stages of grief for her waist-length hair, that she was most likely working her way through. I was forty-nine so although she was half my age her pain was double, just because she was young. My heart missed a beat as I contemplated the idea that she might be ill. I watched and sent her distant healing. In the end I couldn't watch for another second without giving some comfort. I went and sat beside her and asked if she was doing treatments (a nice way of asking if someone has cancer, without bringing the word 'cancer' into either of your space!). Her answer was like a brilliant sun bursting through the clouds after a week of storms, "No." I felt my heart lighten instantly. Thank you dear God that this young woman isn't doing a chemo journey. She had a scalp condition. She may have had to wear the wig for years but she was healthy. I felt like my own situation was easier, just from knowing that hers was. I felt so grateful.

On my way out that day I noted another group of women, women who put a big smile on my face. Older women were buying wigs because their own hair was a bit thin, limp or not quite as flattering as it had been in years gone by. I watched as wigs transformed each and every one of them into smart, stylish and attractive more mature women. Well, way to go "Golden Girls", I thought, with a flush of admiration for them. I may be back here again myself one day, but for an entirely different reason!

LOVE IS . . .

WHEN YOUR DAUGHTER KISSES YOUR BALD HEAD AND TELLS YOU THAT YOU'RE BEAUTIFUL!

FIRST CHEMOTHERAPY

It was the morning of November 12th, 2008. I was to start the first round of chemotherapy. Almost! You are already 'in' your chemotherapy days before. About four days beforehand the anxiety starts. During the day, you manage to keep fairly busy and calm. You manage to semi-block thinking about the impending challenge. The only hint that something majorly unpleasant lies in wait is the edginess you feel—your fuse may be slightly shorter than usual and you may have difficulty focusing on tasks. Basically, no matter how hard you try, you can't think about anything else.

If you somehow manage to keep a semblance of normality about you during the day, once darkness falls and you face the long night, you'll be only too well aware of what you are facing as the fear factor surfaces. Even if you sleep, it's fitful, restless, shot with heart-pounding moments and every muscle in your body is tense. You pass the night in and out of semi-sleep. In spite of the fact that you haven't slept well, the first rays of morning light are welcome.

I really understood where I was 'at' the night before the chemo treatment, when I stood at my kitchen counter and took the steroid tablets, 1,2,3 . . . 8,9,10. Done! I hated the idea of taking so many steroid tablets but I knew they were a necessary evil.

Now here's a revelation. One would imagine that with the level of anxiety in the four days preceding the chemo treatment that I'd be completely 'out of it' on the morning of the treatment itself . . . but no, I wasn't. I woke up and was simultaneously surprised and pleased to feel a sense of relative calm wash over me. It was D-day. Being nervous was pointless at this stage and wasn't going to change anything. Logic kicked in too. I was sick, help was on hand, in the form of chemotherapy, so I decided to embrace it, as best I could, rather than reject the experience.

It was an important comfort to pack all the right things for a full day at the hospital (8 a.m. till about 6 p.m.). I normally packed:

o A book
o A journal/notebook and pen
o My iPod, with podcasts, music and meditation at the ready
o Photographs of loved ones
o Cards that had been sent to me with wonderful energy
o My favourite aromatherapy oil. Sometimes there can be a smell that's unpleasant, for you, or no smell at all and you can adjust your environment to something pleasing, restful and reminiscent of home with your oils
o All relevant medical papers. I highly recommend just bringing your 'famous folder'

(see pages 213-214) with all your medical history (for this illness) to date in it

o Your phone. You will send and receive messages and calls from loved ones throughout the very long day

o Some money, there will be a cafeteria

o Sanitizer, wipes, tissues

o Food for the day. Food is served at the hospital but if you have preferences or are following a special healthy diet then bring your own. I normally brought soup, a wholegrain sandwich, vegetable sticks, fruit, dried fruit, a salad, lots of water and tea

o I always brought two china mugs, one for me and one for any friend that might visit!

o Consider the following before choosing what to wear:

  ✓ You'll be wearing what you choose for the entire day, whether you are sitting or lying down. I once made the mistake of wearing a sweat-shirt with a hood, which was so uncomfortable later when I lay down and was trying to sleep

  ✓ I suggest a layered look. If you wear a cardigan or sweatshirt over a t-shirt, remember that the sleeves of the sweatshirt need to be loose enough to slip easily over your IV needle, if you feel too hot or cold. The IV needle could be positioned anywhere from your elbow to your knuckles!

✓ I found pashminas to be very useful in that they could be easily thrown over my shoulders, my feet, my pillow or wherever necessary

✓ I feel that loose, comfortable elastic-waisted 'bottoms' are best. Think about it, you'll be either sitting or lying all day. You'll have to take the IV stand with you to the bathroom and eat with it too, so in theory, you'll only have full use of one hand for the duration, therefore, struggling with zips and buttons may present a challenge

✓ I found slip-on shoes, like clogs, crocs or flip-flops to be easiest to manage on the many trips from bed to bathroom, remembering again that lacing or buckling a shoe would not have been easy with one hand

✓ I always wore socks as the air-con can get cold, as the day wears on, in an enclosed room

o Needless to add, like everything else in life, you learn as you go along and having made mistakes with what I brought and didn't bring to the unit with me, with how I packed my bags and where I positioned my gear for the day, I got it right in the end. I learned that it was important to pack the food in one bag, the items I'd like to have immediate and continual access to in a second bag and the rest of the stuff in a third bag.

Considering the notion of chemotherapy is basically an unpleasant one, the experience at this unit was as pleasant as such an experience could be. The nurses and doctors were all friendly (but matter-of-fact), helpful and consummate professionals. They inspired confidence.

The chemo unit had eight beds arranged around the walls of the room, with the nurse's station in the centre, in full view of every bed and patient. I chose a bed and settled in for the day.

I handed over my papers and the process began. A nurse set me up with an intravenous needle—quite a sophisticated looking piece with a lid on top. I was later to learn the function of the lid. Finding a vein, that first day, was straightforward because my veins were still in good shape and hadn't yet collapsed due to chemotherapy. It's a good idea (in hindsight!) to have the needle inserted into your less dominant arm, in other words, if you are right-handed, then have the needle positioned in your left arm. Let's face it, if you are going to have full use of only one arm/hand for the entire day, then at least let it be the arm you usually use.

We all (Champs receiving chemotherapy that day) took our turns getting 'set up'. Bags of liquid (happily all colourless!) were hung up and replaced all day long.

I was so impressed with the huge care that was taken (checking and double-checking) that the bags of Chemo 'cocktail' had my name and details on them, before connecting me.

I've had a life-long 'anti' to drugs and substances of every kind. It took huge amounts of visualization, meditation, self-talk, replacement of thoughts, affirmation and whatever else I could think of, to try to welcome these chemicals into my body, to see them as my friend, to perceive them as my healers and to think of them as saving me as opposed to destroying me.

Contrary to popularly held opinion, the chemo day itself is not actually a difficult day as such, once a suitable vein has been found. Chemo day is best described as a very, very long day.

You are in the one place in the world where everyone in it completely understands your situation— the doctors, the nurses, the patients, the technicians, everyone. It's a place where it's okay not to wear a wig, it's okay to be pale, thin and gaunt; it's a place where, for a day, you can allow yourself to be tired, unwell, struggle and even feel a bit sorry for yourself; it's a day when you don't have to try to be, or seem to be, any stronger, healthier or well than you really are; it's a day that's all about you, your treatment programme, your drugs and your reaction to those drugs; it's about resting, giving your body a chance and taking time out from the busy world of 'everyday'; it's a day to meet other women who are in the same position as you, with the same type of cancer, doing the same treatments with the same drugs and, most likely, the same side-effects. These women have had the same surgeries too and face the same, or very similar, challenges, pain, frustrations, fears and exhaustion. There is comfort in being amid this sameness. It gives validation and hope.

I was connected to the drip all day so whether I sat, lay down, walked around, ate or went to the bathroom, the drip came with me. The monitor made a sound I'll never forget and will always be a trigger for me . . . click, phinggg. That sound is entrenched in my memory.

The drugs that constituted the get-well cocktail were Taxol and Carboplatin. I was allergic to both and even to the plaster that held the needle in place in my vein. My body was screaming 'no' to chemicals and substances. I needed to work on this.

I lay down and did some breathing exercises, breathe in "relax," breathe out "release," over and over, till my breathing calmed and my heart-beat returned to normal. I worked on visualization— seeing the drugs as little pink balls with open mouths swimming up my veins and gobbling up all the cancer cells (black, of course!) in sight, before making their way down the opposite side of my body, out through the soles of my feet and back to mother earth. I meditated. Finally, I fell into an exhausted sleep to the hum of the monitor . . . click, phinggg.

My own feeling when my body shows signs of allergy is that my body is saying "no," rejecting and shouting "Hey, this doesn't suit me, stop." Now, I had to delete a lifetime of my personal logic and behavior and adopt conventional medicine's response—shoot a different drug into my vein to counteract the allergy . . . that's what the lid on the IV needle was for! I can't tell you how much I worked on myself in order to come to terms with this way of dealing with an allergy. But, I did. We continued.

This is not a day you spend alone, with a needle in your arm and a drip as a constant companion. The nurses are over and back to you all day, adjusting your monitor, hanging up new bags of 'cocktail' and checking on you. The social worker drops in to see how you and your family are coping and whether assistance, on any level, is required. She'll give you visualization/meditation CD's, books, pamphlets and whatever you need. In some cases, her most valuable contribution is that she listens. The oncologists do their rounds and you can ask questions about what, in medical terms may seem insignificant but, for you, today, may be huge—and you will get answers to allay your worries. The oncologists don't stay long and they are not needed. What you need today, the nurses do so very well. There is so much help available.

Most likely your partner, family member or close friend will stay at the unit with you for the entire day. They may not sit by your bed all day and it's not necessary. You may want some quiet time to meditate, read a little, send a few text messages to the dear 'sisters' who care so deeply and wish you well. Your partner can take breaks and go to the coffee shop to meet his own friends, who in turn come to support him. He may want to catch up on some work with a lap-top, or make phone-calls. He may just want to take some time to relax—don't forget that his life has been turned upside-down too. He is doing more, helping more, worrying more and yes, he really is tired too.

Sometimes friends come by. That's wonderful because a chat and a good laugh really lighten the day and help to speed up the long hours.

Because of my allergic reaction, I was the last one to leave the unit that day, at 7 p.m. I wasn't fed up about the length of time, but rather, I was relieved to note that great care, and every possible precaution, was being taken to ensure that I was well enough to go home, before releasing me.

So, how did I feel at the end of my first day of chemo? I was majorly relieved to have started treatment at last. I felt happy that constructive help was underway. I was delighted that there was no pain or discomfort (that day!)—apart from having a large needle in my arm all day! I felt weary as opposed to tired. It was so refreshing to get out in the open space of the car park and breathe fresh air, after being cooped up in the chemo unit, connected to a machine, all day. I was more than happy to be on my way home.

Knowing that I was attending the best hospital in the land; that I was under the watchful eye of a dream-team of oncologists and the staff that had, quite clearly, been hand-picked; that I was a name and not just a number and that I had access to the unit and team 24/7 all helped to inspire great confidence and calm. I felt that I was not alone, that I was in very experienced and capable hands. I felt safe and that the professionals to whom I was entrusting the task of returning me to good health (and ultimately, saving my life) were so capable, experienced and dedicated. So far, so good!

CHEMOTHERAPY AND ME . . .

SIDE-EFFECTS

Lots of people mistakenly think that the day you receive chemotherapy is a dreadful, pain-ridden, physically challenging day, but it's not, at least, it wasn't for me.

What was tough (understatement!) was the period of time (which usually started two days after the administration of the drugs) between when the side-effects took over till they faded, which took between five to ten days.

Once I felt the pains and other side-effects setting in and stealing all over my body, I knew it was starting and I braced myself for another journey to hell and back. It felt like I had been pushed off the window-sill of the world. From that moment on, I was no longer part of real life, or the world around me. I was unable to connect with it or function as a normal part of it. I retreated into a world of pain, discomfort, inability to sleep, dulled and dazed senses, deadened emotions and physical movement. The entire duration of the side-effects felt like one long block of time as opposed to five to ten endless separate days and nights. After some of the rounds of chemotherapy, when the side-effects wore off, I walked around my home as one would do after returning from a vacation. I honestly felt that I hadn't been physically present at all and had missed out on an entire block of time in my own life and that of the life and activities of my family.

I'd slowly move around the house, from room to room, reacquainting myself with everything, noting changes, enjoying folding a little laundry here, opening a cupboard there, checking a long list of unanswered e-mails, returning calls to dear people that I may or may not have spoken to while I was in the 'trance' of the side-effects. I had only vague and confused memories of events that had occurred during my 'absence'.

Could anyone or anything have prepared me for this? No, definitely not. No amount of words, explanations or reading could have conveyed the intensity, the sensations or the endurance necessary to come out the other side of this experience.

It was clearly explained at the oncology unit, before treatments commenced, that there would be no point in asking anyone else who had cancer and done chemo, even if they had the same cancer and the same chemotherapy drugs as I was about to have, as each person and everyone's body reacts differently. This I found to be true but on the other hand, the side-effects suffered, by most of the women I spoke to, at the unit, who had received the same 'cocktail' as I had, were very similar in type, intensity, duration and impact to mine.

I had six rounds of chemotherapy in all, three weeks apart. The drugs administered were Taxol and Carboplatin. The side-effects for each round were more or less the same, varying only in intensity and or duration, from round to round. Generally speaking, the side-effects lasted longer and were more difficult to cope with as the treatments progressed—but I did live to tell the tale and no matter how hard it was, I managed and was well enough (barely!) three weeks after each treatment to return for more!

The side effects were:

o Intense and extremely severe bone pain
o Abdominal pain
o Complete constipation
o Delayed short-term memory
o Poor hand-eye co-ordination
o Blurred vision
o 'Fuzzy' brain (chemo brain)
o Hearing impairment
o Difficulty walking due to the pains in my legs and severely so in my feet
o Hair loss—every hair on my body
o My breathing was affected
o I could feel the pressure on my heart
o My lymph nodes ached
o Weight loss
o Every cell in my body felt like it was affected, to a greater or lesser degree.

The side-effects start slowly and it feels like they invade every cell in your body. Strong pain killers dulled the pain but never took it away completely. The period of side-effects was almost unbearable, to the point where I thought, on the third round of treatment, that the chemo itself might just finish me off.

On two occasions I was too weak, and my immune system was too low, to go ahead with more treatment, so it was delayed till my immune system got strong enough to continue.

I was very fortunate never to have had nausea or vomiting. I was truly grateful to have been able to eat normally, which in turn helped me to stay as strong as possible.

My whole look changed to the point that at times people passed me and didn't recognize me. At other times I could clearly see that they had only recognized me because my daughter was standing beside me! It takes getting used to others not recognizing you, not to mention you not recognizing yourself! I can assure you that in time, when you are healthy, well and strong again, you will look like your own wonderful self.

It's hard to put into words the effort it took and the impact on my body, of working so hard, to recover from each round of chemo, being barely strong enough again in time to start all over again. It might be like being run over by a bus every three weeks. The difficulty being that each time you start again from a weaker position—lower immune system, thinner, weaker and possibly challenged spirits too.

I saw the time between receiving a dose of chemotherapy and coming out the other side, post the side-effects, as 'time off the world'. I don't mean that as a time to relish or enjoy. No, but whether you plan it, or not, it is a time of introspection, growth and evolvement. There's a very real possibility that you are too unwell, tired and overwhelmed to consciously think about your life in any serious way, but don't worry, awareness floods in all by itself and lessons are learned anyway. It's a time of healing and growth, not just on a physical level.

You may feel that days and days are passing by and you aren't doing anything . . . but you are working so hard to heal, recover, survive and stay alive. Focus on what you are able to do and forget the rest for now. Even if you only manage to get up, shower, see your child off to school, your partner off to work, walk your dog, or whatever, that's something too and in time, you'll be able for more. You need to get up every day even if you have to go back to bed later. You must do it for yourself and for the people around you. It sends your body a 'get up and live' message.

Chemotherapy is such a strange phenomenon, it heals and destroys at the same time and you really do feel the impact of both functions in your body as treatments progress. It strips you down to your very soul. Tears become part of your daily routine, lots of them and often. There were times when I was so spaced from pain that I cried my eyes out and sobbed endlessly. There were times when the concept of making it to the end of this journey seemed out of my reach. You could be forgiven for thinking, at times, that it's never going to end. Thankfully, everything in the Universe changes all the time, so no matter how difficult and terrible your situation is, it will change and most likely, for the better. So, with that in mind, it's obvious that the only way to manage this journey is one day at a time.

Stick with as much of your wellness programme as you are capable of, on as many days as possible, for you. If you can't do everything every day (and most likely you won't be able to; I know that as hard as I tried, I wasn't able), just do whatever feels right for you on that particular day. You could choose from the following ideas:

o Walking
o Organic vegetable juices
o Healthy, fresh, organic and non-processed food
o Contact friends and family
o Laugh, sit down, nap, do nothing!
o Lots of hugs
o Meditation, sitting still, being mindful, listening to music to still the soul
o Breathing exercises
o Reiki or yoga

I wanted my children to see that this wasn't too big for me, that I could handle it and come out the other side. I wanted them to see that this is what

I thought, how I felt, what I expected to happen, what I planned towards and how I intended to live, no matter how hard things got, or how unlikely it seemed from the outside looking in. I wanted to portray illness (in particular, this illness—cancer) as something we can recover from in a positive way (at least that was my plan!). When I felt really bad, and looked even worse than I felt, I'd say "I'll feel a lot better tomorrow."

When you feel totally frustrated with the side-effects, your inability to function 'normally' and the isolation from your regular life, treat yourself gently and recognize your situation for what it is, a journey to vibrant health, a new and cancer-free life. It will take time. Recovery is slow. Do not be discouraged, there is a purpose to all this. All will be well in time, you'll see—you may have to wait just a little bit longer.

COPING WITH THE SIDE EFFECTS . . .

PAIN CONTROL

I've always been astonished at the number of people who overdose at night—take too many pain-killers, a sleeping pill too many or a tranquilizer too much. I could never quite fathom it . . . not until now, that is. Chemotherapy taught me a thing or two and dealing with agonizing and endless pain was one of them. There were times when I would have done almost anything to be free of pain . . . and I would have been satisfied with five pain-free minutes!

It didn't take me long to figure out how highly dangerous it is to leave your pain medication within easy reach as you sleep. Big mistake! The level of pain I was in at times led me to understand what it must be like to be drug-dependent and in need of a fix. You'd be willing to do almost anything for those few blissful pain-free moments.

So, what I did was take pain medication before getting into bed. At the same time, I'd leave another correctly measured 'portion' of pain control ready in a glass, within walking distance of my bed. In this way, there was no question of me, in a moment of desperation and inability to take the pain, reaching out in the dark and grabbing **anything** to relieve the pain.

I found that as well as having the next dose of pain medication at the ready that I also needed a clock. Yes. I'd have a quick look at the clock and check if it was time to take another dose, or not.

Sometimes the pain relief would last only ninety minutes, leaving me with another one hundred and fifty minutes to wait till I could medicate again . . . that's a heck of a long time to wait when you are in pain and everyone else is asleep!

WHEN I'M IN PAIN . . .

LIFE'S LIKE A MOVIE

Four long days had passed since I'd received the first chemotherapy treatment and I was still in really bad shape. I was in severe pain, totally constipated, my brain felt fuzzy, my hand-eye co-ordination wasn't in sync, my vision was blurred, my short-term memory wasn't up to speed and I'd never felt as tired in my life.

My mobile phone was broken and needed to be replaced. Wanting to choose a phone that would best suit my needs, I decided to make the trip to the phone shop at my local mall. My husband and daughter accompanied me as I wasn't capable of driving or going it alone. Naturally, waiting till a day when I was in better physical shape would have been wiser, but remember, this was my first treatment and I had no idea for how many more days the side-effects would last, so today seemed as good a day as any to go—I had no guarantee that I'd feel any better tomorrow.

Even slow walking was a challenge. We made our way to the phone-shop. Our turn came and we sat in front of the rep. I was at my best to focus on what he was saying. Even though I could hear him, my brain wasn't processing the information. Just sitting upright took all of my effort and energy.

The rep looked at me as it became clear that I wasn't quite keeping up. My look was blank.

He continued to sell with the utmost courtesy. When he pulled the fourth phone from the box, assembled it and set it up for my inspection, I just said "Yes, I'll take it." I had no idea what I was purchasing, it would do. I couldn't go on for another nano-second.

Later, I sat down heavily on a bench outside the shop, while my daughter and husband went about other errands. I knew I wouldn't be able to keep up. As I sat down on the seat, so physically small but feeling as heavy as an elephant, tears stole away from my eyes.

Through the blur of tears I looked left and right of me. I saw people rushing about, intent on the business of shopping. I was so slowed up that their movements, in comparison, seemed even swifter. I wondered if I'd ever again, in this life-time, manage to cope with the mall; whether I'd ever again be able to rush around and do my errands; whether I'd ever again be a fully functioning member of the real world. Right now I had serious doubts.

I sobbed, cried and released weighty sighs. I looked around again and knew I just couldn't come even close to coping or participating in the real world. Tears gushed faster when the penny dropped. "Yes, it's as if life is a movie . . . and I'm no longer in it." More serious sadness welled up inside me when I pondered the question "Will I ever be part of the movie again?" I suddenly felt overwhelmed with exhaustion, so incapable and very old indeed. I still had to figure out from where

I'd muster the energy to walk the short distance back to the car. Let the movie roll on without me, I thought, because for the moment, I just can't keep up.

MY LIFE NOW . . .

NEUTROPENIA

You might ask, "What's that?" Your white blood cells may drop very low during chemotherapy. When the white blood cells fall below a certain level you have a condition called neutropenia. During this period of time, you are at high risk of infection.

It is imperative to stay infection free during the months of chemotherapy. Not only are you at high risk of infection when your white blood cell count is so low but, should you be unfortunate enough to develop an infection, your body may be less able to fight it.

During chemotherapy your blood will be tested and monitored frequently so you'll know how strong your immune system is and what your white blood cell count is.

Before setting off on the chemotherapy journey, a chemotherapy nurse will explain, in detail, the measures and steps you'll need to take in order to protect yourself from infection for the duration of your illness. Don't be alarmed, it's not complicated, just basic hygiene. You'd be amazed at how simple precautions can keep you so well during such a major illness. I managed to keep myself devoid of infections of every kind for eight months, so these guidelines work and are worth heeding.

You won't be able to stop your white blood cell count from dropping so you'll do your utmost to avoid infection. Do your very best to keep your skin, mouth, digestive tract and genital area extra clean and avoid injury, cuts, scrapes and nicks. In general, avoid activities that might risk injury.

Wash your hands often and always do when your return home from having been out anywhere, before preparing or eating food (anything) and after using the bathroom. Keep your hands away from your face. Sanitize all the time—when you come out of stores, when you touch buttons in a lift, hold the rail on a stairs or escalator, touch handles on public doors, or shake hands with people (try to avoid hugging, hand-shaking, and cheek-kissing if possible). Avoid being in crowded public places like theatres, cinemas, supermarkets, schools, lecture halls, public transport and swimming pools. Avoid handing animal waste and wash your hands thoroughly after petting an animal. Keep away from anyone who is sick or has been vaccinated recently.

You can help things along by wearing gloves when washing dishes or gardening. It's important to protect your skin with sunscreen when outdoors.

It's best not to eat raw meat, eggs, fish or seafood.

I didn't visit my dentist or hygienist during treatments. Consult with your oncologist if you need to see either.

Here are a few ways you can prepare for an infection free time:

o Place anti-bacterial soap beside all sinks in your home
o Have sanitizer in your bag, in your car and anywhere else you think you'll need it
o Don't share any personal care products, or towels (not even kitchen towels) with anyone else
o Keep your nails short and no false nails
o Rinse your mouth with bicarbonate of soda and salt after every meal and whenever you brush your teeth—it keeps mouth ulcers at bay
o Drink lots of water every day, at least 1.5 litres
o Eat a healthy diet, it will keep you strong.

If during the neutropenia phase your temperature rises (above 38*C/100.5*F), get in touch with your doctor immediately, it may mean that you have an infection. If an infection is not treated quickly it can be more difficult to get it under control later. Common signs of infection would be a burning sensation when urinating or urinary frequency, any redness or swelling of skin, cuts or sores, coughing, sore throat, fever, chill, sweating, diarrhea, vaginal discharge, mouth sores, any such symptom or feeling unwell in any way.

The high-risk time is about between seven to fourteen days after you receive a chemo treatment. Sometimes it can take up to ten days to fully recover from a chemo treatment and this then brings you right up to the 'danger' period with your immune system, when you need to be extremely cautious and careful. It can be a bit disappointing going from possibly ten days of chemo side-effects, right into low immune system days, for a further seven to fourteen days. Then, it's back for another round of chemo. You may feel that you haven't had any break, have hardly been out and you haven't had any fun or time to enjoy in between sessions. Your joy for the moment will have to be that you are infection free, staying strong, coping well with your treatments and that you are well enough to go ahead with the next round of chemotherapy! Remember that anything that is part of getting better is a reason to be grateful and joyful. There will be plenty of time later for enjoying and having fun, when you are healthy again.

Enjoyment for now has to be in open spaces where there are no crowds and where there is lots of fresh air. It's a small price to pay for staying well and infection-free.

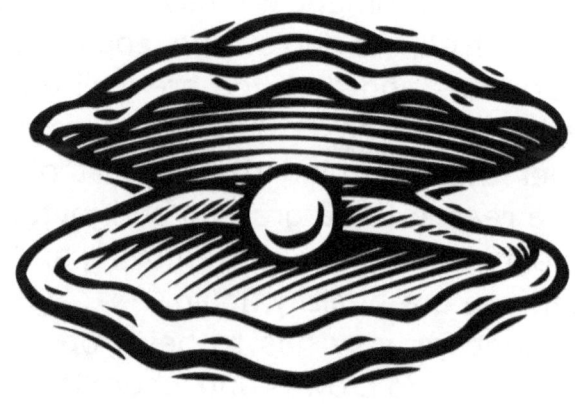

Create something beautiful from a
challenge.

GRAN-ISMS

My Gran died in 1980, when I was twenty. We had always been very close and had so much in common. I loved her and missed her deeply when she passed away.

Over the years I felt her closeness and her 'energy' nearby, mostly when times were challenging. I couldn't see her but I could sense her presence and was always moved to tears when I felt her energy around me.

Gran was with me from the start of the cancer journey until long after I had well and truly healed. Sometimes I could hear her voice. She didn't say a lot but I heeded and acted on all her sound 'gran-isms'.

In the early days I often felt her presence near my bed as I tried to sleep. It was reassuring to know she was watching over me. I knew I was not alone.

She told me to be sure to get out of bed whenever I could. I did, every day of the journey. Sometimes I had to return to bed a few hours later but I started each and every day like a 'real' day—showering, dressing and putting my make-up on, as I would have done, had I not been ill.

At one point, early in the journey, the road ahead seemed endless and I wondered whether, physically, I'd be able for it. I cried, "I'm only on day five of my first treatment, I've got one hundred and eighty five days to go," (just till the end of the treatments, not counting recovery time!) but Gran didn't let me away with that! "You are able," she announced firmly. My healer friend, Dorit, knowing that emotionally and spiritually I was in a strong place, asked me to change Gran's message to "My body is able." From this grew the affirmation that I said so many times a day throughout the months of surgeries, treatments, recovery and right up till today "My body is healthy, well, able and strong. The surgeries, chemotherapy and alternative treatments are healing my body to perfect, vibrant and lasting health." Today I just say "My body is healthy, well, able and strong."

She advised me to have fresh flowers in the house until I was well again. What a wonderful idea—the flowers cheered me up, reminded me of my Gran and, for me, represented summer, full life and vibrant health.

On another occasion she asked me not to let myself 'go'. By that she meant that I should keep myself well groomed and neat. That was sound woman to woman advice. I decided that even if I was going to spend the best part of the next year 'off the world' that I'd do it as stylishly as possible! On a day when I felt a little stronger I bought several stylish leisure-suits, socks and t-shirts in all kinds of fun colours and any other items that I felt would, even under the current circumstances, help me to feel as feminine, stylish and smart as possible.

I was deciding which shoes to wear to the hospital for the first round of chemo. I wasn't sure whether to wear my leather clogs or crocs. Gran's voice, loud and clear over my shoulder, indicated "The leather ones." I laughed out loud . . . that would have been so like her . . . look smart and stylish at all times . . . even in hospital, at the chemo unit!

I clearly recall one night closing the world out as I locked my bathroom door. I already had the 'chemo' look, I felt as weak as a kitten, was as pale as a ghost, my head was completely bald and I felt truly sorry for myself. Resting my arms on the counter-top, I hung my head over the sink and sobbed. I was running on empty. Then I heard her voice say "Stand up straight." It wasn't just "Stand up" but "Stand up straight!" I got it. She was watching me feeling sorry for myself, drowning in self-pity, sinking fast into the illness, in mind as well as body and she came to save me. I did stand up straight, with a smile on the face that I no longer recognized as my own—I felt so safe knowing that she was watching and refused to let me collapse under the weight of the challenge.

Sometimes on chemo days, when the afternoon wore on, other Champs had gone home and I was alone for a time in the deathly stillness of the ward, I would sense her presence. Her energy felt so overwhelmingly loving, tears would just flow and I felt sure that no matter how long it took, that I would be alright.

When everything was over, she reminded me about flowing with things.

Once she asked me to remember everything I'd learned from her while she was alive.

During challenging times in life we are never alone. The souls, energy, love, (call it what you will) of loved ones who have passed away are here with us. They support, guide and love us when we most need it. We can call on them and ask for the help that we need.

HELP FROM
'THE OTHER SIDE' . . .

AFFIRMATIONS

Affirmations are positive sentences we repeat again and again, either out loud or in our minds, with a view to changing our thinking, our attitude, our behavior, our health or some element of our lives that we feel needs to be worked on at this moment in time.

Our subconscious is **unable** to distinguish between truth and falsehood so it believes whatever it is fed. Whatever you nourish your mind with, it believes is fact and responds to accordingly. You, and only you, are in charge of what goes into the 'inbox' of your brain, so choose carefully!

Okay, so that's the theory! What does it really mean for you? What did it mean to me when I was on the cancer journey? Did it work?

Saying affirmations put me in the driver's seat of a situation that otherwise felt out of control. Here was something that I could take charge of. By saying the affirmations over and over I began to believe that what I was saying was true. My affirmations never failed to boost my energy level, put a spring in my step, help me to see things differently and improve my overall feeling of wellness.

Here are some examples of affirmations that really worked well for me:

1. "My body is healthy, well, able and strong. The surgeries, chemotherapy and alternative treatments are healing my body to perfect, vibrant and lasting health."

On a day when I had suspicions that the chemo itself might just finish me off, saying affirmation number one convinced me otherwise.

2. "My name is Dee and today I choose to balance my CA125 (ovarian cancer marker) level. My body is a perfect healing organism and so it is."

When I saw that my CA125 level was rising consistently, never staying the same or dropping, I said affirmation number two. It helped me to see the cancer marker as a number, but that my body was a perfect healing organism in spite of that and, in time, all would be well again.

3. "The nerve endings in my hands and feet are in perfect working order."

Throughout the treatments, and for at least six months afterwards, I had Raynaud Syndrome, in my feet in particular—buzzing/ numbness/pain. Each time I put my feet on the ground was a staunch reminder of where I had come from and of the destruction (as well as healing) the chemo had caused. Doctors assured me that it could take a very, very long time for it to disappear, if at all. I was led to understand that whatever condition my feet were in, six months post-treatment, I'd most likely be left with for the rest of my life. Well, I guess the doctor who said that had never heard of affirmations! One year later I can attest to the fact that my feet are in perfect working order and pain free. If my feet hurt, it's usually when I'm very tired—but then, most people's feet hurt when they are tired!

4. "I am healthy, happy and healed."

On days when thoughts of illness or fears and negative memories surfaced, or when I felt like bouncing with joy I felt so well, I said the above affirmation. Each word held its own value and weight. Each word stated where I was, how I felt and the type of energy I chose to allow into my space.

5. "I'm a cancer survivor."

On days when I felt exceptionally proud of my achievement or when I didn't feel 100% physically well I'd say "I'm a cancer survivor." I'd feel, that's it, it's a fact, nothing can change that!

Make up your own affirmations in accordance with your needs, just remember to:

o Keep them short
o In the present tense
o Refer to your goal
o Avoid the use of negatives
o They must be only about you and your needs
o Be specific
o Say them as many times as possible every day.

For example:

1. My body is letting go of cancer in all its shapes, sizes, forms and expressions.
2. My body is rejecting, uprooting and letting go of all cancer tumours and cells now.

I found it was most effective to say these affirmations first thing in the morning and as often as I remembered throughout my day. There were days when climbing the stairs felt like scaling Mount Everest. I can tell you that the more frequently I said my affirmations, the easier moving around became, the stronger I felt and the more positive my outlook was. They worked magically.

If you have difficulty remembering to say your affirmations then say them first thing in the morning, last thing at night, (saying them last thing at night was hugely important to me because these thoughts and words were then what my subconscious had all night to ponder!), when brushing your teeth, when taking your daily walk, before and or after you eat, every time you are in pain or discomfort, when you feel you are not coping, or when you feel tearful and overwhelmed. You will know.

MY OWN AFFIRMATIONS . . .

DOCTORS

There are good doctors and there are great doctors. A good doctor does his job to the best of his ability. A great doctor listens, looks at you when you are speaking and treats you and every element of your relationship with the utmost respect—your body, your health, your fears, your questions, everything. Medicine is a way of life for great doctors, they are naturals and they are passionate about what they do.

Your doctor is your staunchest ally, when you find a great one, as your work your way back from death's door to vibrant health. I was fortunate enough to have found myself in the hands of the most outstanding, experienced, skilled and totally professional doctors and surgeons, 99% of the time. I entrusted my life into their very capable hands with the utmost confidence. I didn't just think they were the very best, I knew it.

Great doctors deserve our endless and undying gratitude above all else. They give so much of their time, effort and energy to serve a huge volume of sick people, day in and day out. They work endless hours to cure us, return us to quality health and extend our lives.

Do you have 110% (that's not a miss-type!) confidence in your medical team? You need to feel relaxed and comfortable with your doctors, you need to feel free to ask questions, voice your worries and say what you think. If you don't click with your doctor, or if you don't like your doctor's attitude, his outlook, his approach, how he speaks to you or if for any reason, your gut feeling tells you that this is not the right doctor for you, you should find another one. The road to recovery is long and you need to feel very comfortable with your doctor. He needs to believe in your full recovery as much as you do. If you can find a doctor that gives you the feeling that he is working 'with' you, as opposed to 'on' you, you'll be truly fortunate.

No one knows your body better than you do. What feels right to you and for you? Learn to trust yourself as well as your doctor. You are a very important and significant person on your medical team. Be proactive. If your doctor, the treatment, the diagnosis, or anything doesn't feel right to you, if your instincts are screaming "No," you need to listen, make different choices and possibly look for a second opinion. Your doctor will not pay the price if you allow him to bother you off, you will. Insist and persist until you feel completely comfortable with your situation—your life may depend on it.

Don't set your doctor up as a demi-god. Doctors have hugely responsible jobs and do incredible work but they are human beings just like us, who can also have a bad day, feel tired, make mistakes and may not have all the answers.

There were a few incidents on my journey that helped me to understand that 1) I need to listen to my gut feeling and go with whatever feels right for me when it comes to doctors and 2) I need to have a 'buddy' with me at all doctor's visits—someone else to listen, hear and understand any detail I might miss; more importantly, someone who would remember any important information that I might forget, due to feeling unwell in any way.

My gynecologist sent me for a routine vaginal ultrasound in March 2008. A 2.5 cm cyst was found on my right ovary. The gynecologist decided to check it again in May. The result was the same. The only difference this time was that the radiographer recommended, when my examination was done, that the cyst should not be there and needed to be removed. When my gynecologist suggested waiting for another few months to see whether the cyst would vanish all by itself, I passed on the radiographer's recommendation. On hearing this, she leaned over her desk and informed me that the only path open now would be surgery and—wait for this—"Surgery costs money!" I was stunned into silence. Whaaaaaat? I went home and waited. I wondered whose money she was worried about saving. As it turned out, no money was saved at all. My medical insurance provider, the state, my family and I, paid dearly for what I consider to have been her mistake in waiting too long to send me for a biopsy. She was the only bad doctor I met on my entire journey—bad for me, that is!

One of my visits to an oncologist during chemotherapy left me disappointed. When doing chemo, you receive your treatment and then go home to work your way through it. Three weeks later you have a return visit to the oncologist for a check-up. When I proceeded to tell him about the side-effects I'd suffered that round of treatment, he stopped me and said "We know the side-effects." I was stunned by his cold abruptness. Well, hey, I thought, I've struggled through hell and back for three weeks to be well enough to come and tell you how I'm doing and you don't want to listen! Again, I decided on the spot to ensure I'd never come for a check-up on a day when this oncologist was on duty.

These few unpleasant experiences are minor memories compared to the wonderful care I received on my journey from every other doctor. I was so moved when one of the three-team of surgeons came to my room the morning of one of my surgeries, sat on the bed next to mine and chatted to me. He asked about any fears, worries or questions I might have. It made a huge difference.

When the professor who heads the gyne-oncology department would take time to tour the unit and talk to each patient individually, it felt so right. He can't even know the difference that would make.

When my oncologist called one evening at 9.30 p.m. to update me on the results of a CT scan, I knew I was in excellent hands, he really cared.

I found the conventional medical profession, in general, to be skeptical of healers and everything alternative. It didn't take me long to understand why. I feel that this attitude is mainly due to the fact that they know little or nothing about it. Doctors are conventionally trained, they believe in their direction and naturally, they won't recommend or comment on homeopathy, healer's treatments, or any other alternative direction about which they know little or nothing, and that's okay.

For me, healing takes place on all three levels, mind, body and spirit. It's like a three-legged stool. If you lift the stool by one leg, all three legs rise together. Doctors do an outstanding job of removing organs, administering chemotherapy and radiation in order to stop, or slow down, the progress of cancer cells. However, in my opinion, optimal and complete healing cannot take place without all three levels being worked on. Your doctors will work on curing your illness while you will have to work on the other elements of healing yourself.

So what can you do to ensure that you'll be as safe and well cared for as possible? You can insist and persist till you feel you are getting the best care possible but most of all go with what **feels** right for you. If any element of your care doesn't resonate with you, on any level, look elsewhere.

MY DOCTORS . . .

CHEMO PAL

You will, no doubt, be fortunate enough to be surrounded by an extraordinary support circle as you journey though your illness. You may be blessed with a loving partner, understanding children, supportive friends, helpful neighbours and flexible colleagues but there is someone else whose help you will also need. You will need to either join a support group or have a 'chemo pal'.

A chemo pal/support group is essential. Research shows that Champs in a support group or who have a chemo pal do better physically and emotionally. You will be amazed at the beauty of soul and strength of the women. Their capacity to inspire and support one another will profoundly affect the way you view the journey you are on. Their thoughtfulness plus their capacity for empathy will amaze you. Their ability to celebrate the good news and suffer alongside you when there's bad news will touch your heart deeply.

I know some view support groups negatively. They think that these groups are a fancy name for a 'pity party'. I disagree. A woman who is on, or has already completed the journey you now find yourself on, will be a buddy. Buddies share valuable information and they support each other when necessary. They cheer you up and cheer you on, when that's the order of the day. Such support is not just necessary, it's essential.

You might wonder whether it would not drag you down being around 'sick' women but, I can say, from experience, that this is definitely not the case. In fact, I didn't see my chemo pal as being sick—we knew we were sick but somehow we saw beyond that.

I cried and sobbed my heart out on the fifth day of my journey. I came off steroids and completely 'crashed'. I wondered how I'd face the next one hundred and eighty five, or more, days of treatments. That didn't even include at least six further months of recovery time. It all just felt like more than I could handle. It was crystal clear that I'd need a chemo pal or a support group—I needed to be around someone who really understood every detail of this process.

If you do not have a chemo pal, find one. I was fortunate to meet my chemo pal early on my journey. I remember preparing for a treatment and settling into my bed at the chemo unit. I looked down the line of beds on my side of the ward and saw, or should I say, 'recognized' my chemo pal. I looked at her and knew we would be friends and do the journey together.

My chemo pal, we'll call her Lorna, was on her second 'tour' with cancer when I started my journey. She understood everything that needed to be understood. She knew what I needed. She knew what helped and what didn't. She knew when to listen and when to advise. Her side-effects carbon-copied mine. I didn't need to describe anything since she felt everything I was feeling.

We accompanied each other to the wig shop to have our wigs washed or styled—we were able to laugh here and there in a situation that wasn't at all funny.

Lorna and I sat in many a queue waiting for our turns to be examined by our oncologist. Of course neither of us chose to sit at the coffee shop at the unit afterwards. No, the unit was a place we both wanted to escape from as fast as our legs could carry us! We both held our breaths when the other waited for blood test results, the tension mounting as we wondered if the 'magic' CA125 level (cancer marker) was up or down this time.

We'd meet on the day of yet another round of chemo, whoever arrived first would save a bed for the other. We'd be equally relieved for each other when a suitable vein had been found and the day's 'performance' could begin. We'd chat, compare 'notes' and catch up until the chemo began to dull our brains, around noon, and we'd fall into a drug induced sleep.

We spoke almost daily on the phone. We listened to detailed descriptions of every pain, ache, sleepless hour, fear, pre and post test/scan/ doctor's visit news.

Lorna warned me in advance of many experiences that I'd have to face a bit further down the tracks. It was helpful beyond measure to be prepared emotionally and have my awareness fine-tuned.

Once we'd finished our treatments we talked about celebrating accordingly, but many weeks went by before either of us was well enough for that. We decided to upgrade our friendship from 'chemo pals' to just 'pals'—it was time to let go of 'treatment talk'. Since then we jokingly tagged ourselves as 'Viking pals' one day and it stuck! It seems appropriate for now since we need to be strong and stay that way.

A SPECIAL CHEMO FRIEND . . .

MAILS FROM THE HEART TO THE SOUL

E-mails from one cancer pal to another are sent from the 'outbox' of the heart, to the 'inbox' of the soul. They can go like this:

o I'm going to a party now. I feel so grateful that I'm well enough to go. I had a good day.
o Thank you for sharing all you have learned and for your good ideas about making lasting changes. Have a healthy and special week.
o I'm doing well and stretching myself more. I seek balance every day.
o I look forward to when you are strong enough to talk. No rush. Sending you love and light.
o How did your treatment go? Breathe in love, life and health. Sending you a hug.
o Have a great day whatever comes your way. We know it's a choice and it's okay to get sad sometimes and then pull ourselves out.
o Wishing you a 'feel good' day today.
o I'm too tired to talk today. My hair has started to fall out in clumps this morning and I'm not even upset. I'm curious to see what I'll look like bald. I think it will be harder for the others than for me. We'll wait and see.

- o I hope your treatment went well yesterday and that you had nice feelings of healing taking place.
- o It was so good to see you yesterday. I count my blessings that we were both well enough to meet.
- o You must be aware of how many lives you are touching and what a huge difference you are making just by doing your own journey—and you can even do it from home!
- o Fear is never gone, just better contained. I feel achy myself in the last couple of weeks and find I do not have a lot of stamina.
- o I've been tired these last few days but I'm so joyful that I've finally learned to say 'no' to others when I'm not able to do something or when I feel tired or need some quiet time or space for me.
- o It was so great talking with you the other day. I was feeling very vulnerable and you really helped me a lot.
- o What's this journey with our physical health and healing about if it's not to enjoy life? I'm done with suffering.
- o You'll soon be six weeks after your surgery and you know how much better one always feels six weeks after any major body event.
- o You'll just have to stay in your own space and keep working on yourself. We can never

'fix' anyone else no matter how hard we try.

o   Another thing I learned on my journey was to see love in a different way.

o   Express clearly what you 'want/need', as opposed to what you 'don't want'. Steer clear of any blame.

o   Do whatever you need to do in order to get well and stay well. Your wellness is the most important thing for you to think about every day.

o   Is there a person, situation, relationship or anything at all, in your life at the moment, that does not resonate with your soul? Some part of something that is currently in your life is keeping you sick. Ask yourself "What am I sick to death of in my life?" There lies the key to your recovery.

o   There can't be anyone around you now who pulls you down in any way or drains your energy. Things are hard enough without extra forces working against you.

o   There will be lots of other lessons, which I will embrace with gratitude, when the time comes.

o   Stay in your own space, do your own journey, plunge forward with your own healing.

o   Take time to think about what you need to do (not what someone else needs to do) in order to get well and stay well and then just do it.

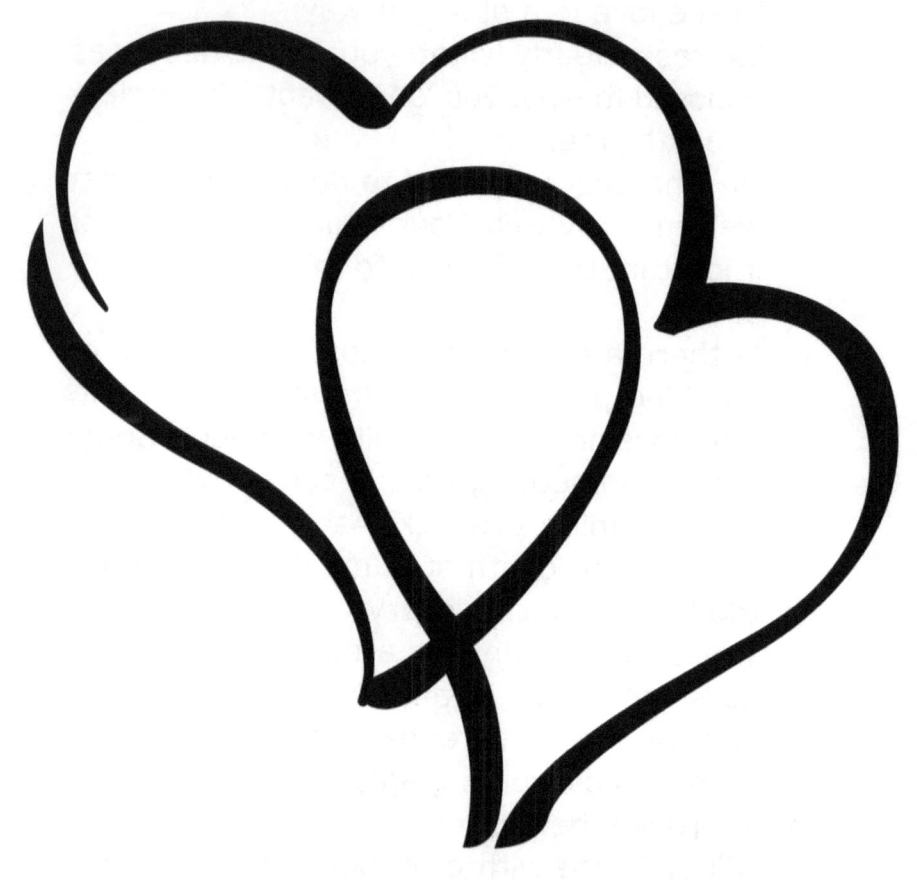

The wisdom of feeling.
Love is all there is.

GENETIC TESTING

"To do a genetic test or not to do a genetic test?" That is the question!

There are many opinions about and answers to this question. None of what I write here is based on medical fact or scientific evidence, it's just my humble opinion. I'll share my personal experience and raise a few questions that will give you food for thought, so that you can consider the subject more carefully and with a more open mind.

It's more than likely that at some stage, during the cancer journey, your oncologist will recommend genetic testing. There are many valid reasons for going ahead with testing.

It could happen that your genetic test results would show that you do not carry the suspect gene, in which case, your chances of developing certain other cancers do not skyrocket to 80%.

There are other reasons to breathe a gigantic sigh of relief if you find you are blessed not to carry the gene, for which you are being tested. The first reason is that you are not in a high risk category yourself for developing further cancer, but also, and more importantly, (at least for me), if you are a mother, it will mean that you will not have passed on such a gene to your beloved daughter. Now that is something to be eternally grateful for.

Let's look at the worst case scenario. You may have tested positive for the gene in question.

Let's say, for example, that you have had ovarian cancer. You would be tested for BRCA1 and BRCA2 genes. If it was discovered that you were a carrier of the guilty gene, your chances of developing breast cancer could jump to 80%. Obviously, at that point, lots of constructive recommendations would be made by the experts, one of them being, a double mastectomy! There are many women, who are members of families where many women have had breast cancer, they do the gene test, are found positive and then go ahead with this surgery. In their case, you can see how wonderful it is that this test is available. You can understand the relief for such women to be able to avail of such preventative measures—the procedures and surgeries could be life-saving.

I had done the fifth round of chemotherapy when I did the genetic test. Fortunately for me, I do not carry the gene. In hindsight, it was not a good idea for me to do the genetic test before I'd completed the chemotherapy and given myself time to recover. If it had been discovered that I was a gene carrier, it would have been too emotionally taxing for me, (I see that now) with all that I was already enduring, to deal with the weight and implications of such a result, at that time.

Every Champ faced with the decision of whether to go ahead with genetic testing, or not, feels differently about it, has her own opinion for specific reasons and needs to choose what she feels is right for her to do at the time, in line with her own personal situation.

One Champ I met, who had the same surgeries and treatments as I had, did the genetic test, discovered she was carrying the gene but decided not to have a mastectomy. Her decision was logical for her. She said she'd been carrying the gene all her life (she was now in her late fifties) without realizing it and hadn't yet developed breast cancer. She also felt that although her chances of developing it were now 80%, she may in reality be in the 20% group that would never develop the disease! She chose not to do preventative surgery, but to live, enjoy and have all the relevant check-ups every six months (mammogram, ultrasound, blood tests and a physical examination by a breast surgeon) and do an MRI scan annually. If she developed breast cancer, she would deal with it, if and when the time came, but not before. She felt comfortable with these choices and they felt right for her at the time.

I know another Champ who has already had breast cancer and ovarian cancer; her Mum died of breast cancer. She has chosen not to be genetically tested to date. You might read this and think she has to be crazy. Having done a cancer journey (and she has done two) I completely understand her fear. She says that if she gets cancer again, she gets it. She has chosen to flow with things as they are. She knows what she can handle and cope with. This is the right decision for her, for now. There is no room for judgment in a situation such as this. Doctors will advise but the ultimate choice and decision about whether to be genetically tested, or not, is hers.

Genetic testing is not just about the woman who does the test, her health and her future. It's about all the women in her entire nuclear and extended family. I would not have even considered not doing the genetic test because I have a daughter, three sisters (including an identical twin) and six nieces. I felt I owed it to them, and not just myself, to go ahead with the test. I have no regrets.

Doing a genetic test is a matter of a simple blood test. Dealing with the results is more complex. It's my personal opinion (and only mine) that genetic testing is a wonderful advancement in medical science. Used in the right way it can prevent illness, pain, suffering, it can extend life, give people choices and is generally a worthwhile procedure. You might wonder why every woman, at high risk of cancer, wouldn't jump at the chance to be genetically tested. Women who think things through before they agree to be tested make the choice that they know they can live with.

Having done a cancer journey and endured surgeries, treatments, tests, scans and more I now understand how fear and your thoughts can affect your mind, your body and your health. Speaking for myself, and only myself, I know that if I was told that I carried the suspect gene and that my chance of developing breast cancer was now 80%,

I imagine that as hard as I'd try to be upbeat, positive, to flow with things and to believe with all my heart that I was healthy, that I'd be fearful (even a little!) and since I know that my thoughts form my reality . . . need I go any further?!

If you find yourself in a situation where you are faced with the option of genetic testing, the bottom line, I think, is to take some quiet time to reflect, read and learn as much as you can about the whole issue, consider and make an informed decision about whether to go ahead or not. If you decide to go ahead, ask yourself sincerely and honestly whether you are sure you can live, in a relaxed and fear-free way, with whatever the results may be. It's a choice—yours.

WILL I?—WON'T I? . . .

SCAN SCARED!

Tears overflow from my heart and down my
cheeks
As I call on all my loved ones who have passed
away, by name.
Please come and hold me now in my time of
dread, terror, fear, anxiety, worry and panic.
Do you know any well-connected angels yet?
Not knowing what's going on inside me is too
much for me now.
Facing another PET/CT doesn't fit.
I've finally figured out what life is about,
How the Universe works,
Uncovered who I am,
Discovered what I was born to do,
Learned so many lessons,
Realized I can make a difference,
And untangled so much wisdom.
I'm ready at last so don't steal my time away,
Don't snatch my chance to live.
Please, I so humbly beg—bestow on me the
treasured time I so soulfully seek.
If all else fails
No matter what the results reveal
Grant me the grace to graciously greet my news
with gratitude,
Acceptance and peace.

I'm not just asking or praying, it's more than
even haggling—
I'm begging and pleading, with the greatest
humility.

Dee

SURGERY

For most Champs, surgery is an inevitable part of the cancer journey. In some cases, it may even mean multiple surgeries. Personally, I'm a great believer in the skills and talents of an experienced surgeon and his team.

On hearing that I'd need a biopsy I was relieved. On learning that there was a possibility that I'd need a full hysterectomy as well, I was crushed, felt dizzy and weak as tears stung the back of my eyes. Whaaat?

I felt I was a young woman who wasn't even pre-menopausal and now, the body I knew, my valued organs and the cycles I'd lived my life around were to be snatched away. My life would change irreversibly. This would take time to absorb.

In fairness, there are many comforting benefits to surgery:

o Surgery removes cancerous tumours and organs
o Surgery is quick and recovery time is short compared to chemotherapy. You will be well enough five days later, even after major surgery, to return home and most likely, within three weeks, you'll be functioning fully and normally again
o When you've had surgery there is a smaller clean-up job, (of rogue cells invisible to the

naked eye of the surgeon, at the time of surgery) for chemotherapy to tackle later

o You can actually feel the physical relief when the cancer has been removed and the symptoms you had prior to surgery (bloating, pain, nausea, loss of appetite and exhaustion) disappear.

In the days preceding surgery it's so important to gather support around you like a cozy blanket on a cold winter's night. Phone-calls, text messages, cards, visits and support of every kind are graciously and gratefully received at this time. You need to know, as well as feel, that you are not alone.

Packing for a surgery is quick and easy because you'll be in a hospital gown and fasting for most of the time you'll be in hospital. So you won't need a lot more than:

o Toiletries and towels
o Easy to slip on footwear: crocks, flip-flops or slippers
o A light-weight dressing-gown
o Reading material
o Notebook or journal & pen
o iPod with music, meditation pieces and podcasts
o A meaningful, lovingly given, symbolic piece for beside your bed
o Family photo or small picture that brings comfort to look at

o Phone
o Aromatherapy oils
o Petty cash
o Your 'famous folder' (see pages 213-214) containing the documents and history of the illness to date
o Loose clothes to wear coming home, remember you'll have a tender scar on your abdomen by then!

You'll be fasting before you arrive at the hospital, which will be the day prior to surgery. Once you've checked in and been shown to your room, you'll be free to have some time alone, which is good. Huge changes lie in wait and one needs time to absorb, internalize and come to terms with this new status.

Some Champs are happy to share a room, while others really need the privacy, stillness and alone-time of a private room, on such a big day. Most likely, the rooming situation in which you find yourself will be perfect for you, including your room-mate, if you should have one. The Universe has a way of working that out in one's favour, on such an occasion.

Throughout the afternoon and early evening you'll be fasting and preparing for surgery— you'll be connected to a drip, medication will be administered, an enema will be performed, nurses will come and talk to you, forms will be filled and every detail will be explained to you.

Personally I was always happy that I was in hospital from the day before surgery. There was nothing to do only lie down, rest and prepare myself for the major physically and emotionally traumatic event of the next day. Best of all was the quietness and stillness. I needed that.

At the end of the day, when everyone has gone home, you are alone. It a time to have a little cry and release fears, anxiety, worry and any other pent-up emotions. It's a good idea to visualize, to meditate, to pray (if you usually do) and to be mindful. I took time to ponder each and every organ that I was about to lose. I thought of how it had loyally served me all my life, how it had functioned without fail for so many years and how I was now ready to let it go with gratitude. I was only too well aware that it was these organs that had brought me my adored children. Letting go of my womb was painful beyond anything I was prepared for. I had never given a thought to how much my womb meant to me, the organ that had protected my growing babies for nine long months. It drew the deepest pain and most endearing memories. I felt so grateful.

Taking a walk down the corridor is a great idea, if you are aware before-hand, that you may be able to see into the rooms of Champs who, today, already had the surgery, that you will have tomorrow! They will not look in good shape, so remember that the body is an amazing healing organism and heals so quickly, including yours! All will be well for them in a day or two and for you too.

We all know that surgery involves wounds, stitches and pain. Fortunately, modern medicine has so many drugs that can ease your symptoms at this time. Being realistic, it's good to accept beforehand that such a major body event can't be totally painless, but don't we all live to tell the tale?!

In the recovery room you'll wake up slowly, hearing muzzy sounds and voices before you can focus enough to see clearly. You'll see your loved ones right beside you and you'll know that surgery is over, you are alive and well. Give thanks.

It's hard to imagine that the morning after major surgery, the bandages are removed, you are helped out of bed to sit in a chair and before you know it you are standing under the shower! Look how fast you are recovering already! You will be shocked at what a truly incredible organism your body is, how much it can endure and still function perfectly for you the next day. Infinite love and gratitude to your beautiful, faithful body, for sure. By the way, removal of the bandage doesn't hurt at all.

On the day pre and post surgery I think having immediate family visit the hospital may be sufficient. Staying in a quieter space may be more beneficial. However, on day two, post surgery, you are more than ready to fill your room with all the beautiful souls that share your journey. It's party time!

Post-op pain is pain that can be handled fairly well with pain-relief. I may be wrong, but my personal experience was that even prescription pain-killers did **not** kill all the pain. They eased the pain, down-graded it and made it more bearable. Once the first two or three days are over, you regain more mobility, flexibility, energy and strength. You will have started eating again and that makes a huge difference. You are on your way at last.

Returning home feels wonderful. The familiarity of home, the joy of being with your family again, the comfort of your own bed, access to your favourite foods, the absence of the busy hospital schedule and the unadulterated joy of having the surgery behind you is enough to boost healing instantly. In the first days at home bending, getting up and down stairs, getting out of bed, staying up for more than a few hours at a time, walking and sitting will be challenging and uncomfortable. As each hour and day goes by you'll find yourself healing, getting stronger and returning slowly but surely to normal function. There is so much joy in that alone.

One week after surgery you'll see the gyne/ oncologist that performed the surgery. You'll have a chance to say how you feel, voice worries, be examined, have your stitches removed and a date will be set for the next leg of your journey. Having stitches removed doesn't hurt!

I haven't met one Champ yet that was upset about having a long scar down her abdomen. In general, Champs look on their scars with pride, after all, they have survived a great ordeal and on a more mundane level, it's all part of getting better, the goal of this journey. I think that being upset about possibly never being able to wear a bikini again wouldn't even be on the radar for most Champs!

There is no lead into your ensuing menopause. One day you are comfortably cruising along within the familiar framework of your menstrual cycle, that you have lived along-side and parallel to for thirty five to forty years. The next day it's as if someone has snipped the connecting cord and it's all over, over-night, all at once.

As much as every woman moans about her pre-menstrual symptoms, period pains and the emotional rollercoaster of it all, month after month, year after year, she enjoys the familiarity, the sameness and the sisterhood of it. I definitely spent many a quiet hour lost in thought before surgery, trying somehow to let go of the only life I'd know since being a teenager. No part of me could image how my new life would be, without the constant companionship of my monthly cycle.

As suddenly as one phase ended, the other was upon me. So, now, here I found myself, floundering at all that I had to face: recovery from major surgery, the end of my menstrual cycle, return to chemotherapy within three weeks of surgery and the full-on onset of menopausal symptoms. Never a dull moment!

Quite frankly, it turned out to be such an easy transition because night sweats and hot flashes paled into complete and total insignificance once I returned to chemo. By the time I'd finished chemo and recovered, all the menopausal symptoms had completely disappeared. I was left trying to decode how it could possibly be that something that had dominated my life for thirty five to forty years could possibly have disappeared and been forgotten without costing me a further thought. It was **over**!

With 'over' came a new-found freedom, a creative surge, a love of the outdoors, an inner surety and accepting embrace of this new phase of my life. No longer having the credentials to part-take in the Young Women's Club, I was now eligible to join the Wise Women's Club!!

LOVE IS . . .

WHEN YOUR TEENAGE SON SWITCHES ROLES WITH YOU AND HE BECOMES THE MUM!

LIBERATION DAY!

January 20th 2009, the day after my full hysterectomy/debulking surgery, was the most liberating day of my life. I can't remember any other day in my life, prior to that date, when I felt such serenity, tranquility, total acceptance and peace.

I lay there in my hospital bed, without eyelashes or eyebrows, without hair, wig or bandana, without my clothes or makeup, and with the large, shapeless, well-worn hospital gown completely drowning my 42kg body. I was pale, skinny and had you passed by my bed that day, you would have been forgiven for assuming that I might not make it!

I was surrounded by dear and special friends, who'd taken time from their own busy lives, to spend all this time with me. There was so much love and compassion in my room that day.

Normally I would not have felt comfortable, not to mention confident, without my clothes and makeup, but that day, I felt free and at peace. This was the day I fully gripped and internalized that we are not 'bodies with souls' but 'souls with bodies'.

I lay there thinking, well, "This is 'me', just as I am. I'm bared down to my very soul now, no trappings or trimmings." It was a life-changing moment for me. Things would never be the same for me again. I actually felt peaceful and free.

THE DAY MY LIFE CHANGED FOREVER . . .

'SISTERS'

"It is not what you have in your life, but whom you have in your life that counts," Anne Mundell.

Someone e-mailed me the following piece one day—I couldn't say it any better than this:

"Time passes, life happens, distance separates, children grow up, jobs come and go, love waxes and wanes, hearts break, parents die, colleagues forget favours, careers end, but . . .

'Sisters' are there no matter how many miles are between you. A girl-friend is never further away than needing her can reach. When you have to walk that lonesome valley and you have to walk it by yourself, the women in your life will be on the valley's rim, cheering you on, praying for you, pulling for you, intervening on your behalf and waiting with open arms at the valley's end. Sometimes they will even break the rules and walk beside you . . . or come in and carry you out. Girl-friends, daughters, granddaughters, daughters-in-law, sisters, sisters-in-law, mothers, grandmothers, aunties, nieces, cousins and extended family all bless our life!

The world wouldn't be the same without women and neither would I. When we began this adventure called womanhood, we had no idea of the incredible joys or sorrows that lay ahead. Nor did we know how much we'd need each other, every day. We need each other still."

So who are these 'sisters'? They are the women in your life who support you, admire you, cheer you on and encourage you. Your 'sisters' are women you know and trust. They inspire you to be the best you can be. You feel comfortable, loved and safe around them. You can talk to them with ease; they listen to your fears; they don't gossip about your secrets and are the epitome of discretion. You feel wonderful about yourself and more confident about trying and doing new things when you are surrounded by your 'sisters'. Your 'sisters' genuinely care and want for you what you want for yourself. They appreciate and love you in spite of the differences. This incredible support can help you to find your direction when you are lost and help you to heal.

No medication will help you let go of past anger, hurt or betrayal the way the support of 'sisters' can. No class, reading or therapy will dissolve your emotional pain and help you to get back on track (and ensure that you stay there) the way the support of this amazing group can, assuming that you are fortunate enough to be surrounded by such 'sisters'. The love, care, support, encouragement, sharing that comes from your 'sisters' is your most valuable asset and treasured possession as you journey through cancer. Hang on to them for dear life! We all need to have such a group around us, it gives our lives meaning, worth and substance.

"Everyone needs a cheering squad," says Susan Jeffers. The role of 'sisters' is to support us, but there is so much more to it than that. Your 'sisters' carry you when life is just too difficult and your legs won't work, because you have fallen down and can't get up or stand alone, at the moment. They carry you till you can function alone again. They never give up on you. They are always there when you need them. 'Sisters' really prove themselves during these challenging times. They are there, no matter what.

If you want strong, supportive, special 'sisters' in your life, then you have to be that kind of 'sister' yourself, long before you think you will ever need them. Then, when your life comes crumbling and crashing down around you, as it does on a cancer journey, they will already be there waiting on the side-lines, to return what they have been receiving from you over the years. It's a give-receive 'round'. What goes around, comes around, and just sometimes, when you least expect it, and sooner than you might anticipate.

MY 'SISTERS' . . .

WHERE ARE YOU?

It can happen that someone close to you (let's call her Louise) just isn't there for you, on this journey, from the very outset. At least, that's how it seems to you, at the time.

When you first share the devastating news of your diagnosis with Louise, you are too numb yourself, at first, to realize that she doesn't appear to quite grip the gravity of your situation and her reaction lacks the expected passion and heart.

As the days pass and you get so much love and support from all quarters, awareness unfolds that Louise is not there for you, at least, not in the way that you need her to be.

Phone calls are all about her and her life; she mostly forgets to ask how you are at all and even when she does, (with the odd prompt from you), she doesn't always wait to hear your answer. It becomes blatantly clear that Louise does not understand what you are going through.

You are in shocked disbelief and complete bewilderment. This could not be happening. Louise is, after all, the one person on the planet whom you thought would be your closest ally on the journey to come. But . . . no!

There's an empty feeling in your heart. The initial pain of the situation gives way to acceptance that she just doesn't know how to be there for you. Of course near and dear ones will tell you that you have enough going on at the moment and to just let go . . . but you can't . . . at least, not just like that . . . not just yet. As the days roll on you realize that you are actually grieving her loss.

In time the emotional pain subsides. You are letting go of a relationship that may never be on the same footing, for you, again. Well-meaning loved ones should not attempt to rush you through this stage, because you need to reflect on the magnitude of your loss and feel the emptiness before you can fill up again.

As you start to adjust to your life as it is, without Louise holding her honoured place, you no longer feel quite as low. You are learning to accept the reality of your situation, as it is.

Finally, you can think of Louise, without sadness. You are able to look around and count the love you have in your life as opposed to the love and support that's missing.

Long after I'd finished grieving, huge awareness came in for me. How could I possibly have missed it? Yes, this whole Louise lesson began to make sense:

o   This was my big lesson in accepting things as they are, or as Byron Katie puts it so nicely, 'loving what is'

o   Louise may have been fearful that what was happening to me could possibly happen to her also one day o She was possibly worried about me and didn't know how to handle it, or know what to say or do

o She was giving what she was able to give and the fact that it wasn't what I needed at the time was irrelevant

o I needed to see and value what she was actually giving and ignore what she wasn't capable of giving

o I needed to accept, with great love and gratitude, all the love that came my way, no matter who was giving it; no matter what shape, size or form it came in; no matter from what level they were giving it; no matter what their motivation; no matter with what frequency; no matter what it was I thought I needed, or wanted at that moment in time, that was different from what I received.

Thank you Louise for the valuable lesson you helped me to learn in acceptance and gratitude. I am now capable of loving and valuing you in what seemed like imperfection, at the time . . . now I know it was perfect and so were you. I need not have wondered where you were, you were there all along, in your own capacity, doing your best, giving all you knew how to give, just being you. Thank you.

I'M DEVASTATED
BECAUSE . . .

GRACE

As a child I often heard the word 'grace' spoken. I wondered what exactly it meant. No one seemed to be able to explain its precise meaning to me. Now I know!

On hearing the mind-blowing diagnosis of ovarian cancer, my voice quivered, my knees knocked together, I felt cold, but inside there was calm—that was grace!

As the surgeries and treatments progressed I lost weight, lost my healthy colour, lost my hair, lost my energy, lost my old life, but I found inner peace—that's grace!

At times when everything seemed just too much to bear, too heavy, too painful and too long, but my soul seemed to float over my body, so I just felt lightness inside and out—that's grace!

Through all the bumps, twists and turns of this journey, when somehow it all felt familiar and I recalled, in the recesses of my sub-conscious mind, that I'd chosen this lesson long before I was born—that's grace!

When I noticed that people in my life were not coping with the illness and instead of them comforting and supporting me, in fact, it was the other way around, I was calming them—that's grace!

When love, support, help, compassion, healing, prayers, good energy and light were sent my way from every continent, every major world religion, even from people whom I'd never met, wave upon wave of serenity flooded my being—that's grace!

When the right healer appeared at the right time, when the most experienced doctors took care of me, when a 'sister' posted me the perfect book for now, when I knew I could easily be dead, but I wasn't, and joy was the only emotion I felt— that's grace!

Grace comes from God, Source, the Universe, the Great Spirit, (the name is not important). Grace is pure, gentle, all-loving, healing, comforting and available to all. You really don't even need to request it, just remain open to the idea that it exists and that you'd be grateful to experience it. Grace comes to you and for you, it becomes part of you, you merge together and find peace.

HOW GRACE TOUCHED MY LIFE . . .

GIFTS

Gifts came in every shape and size. The contents of the packages were always a surprise and brought a smile to my face at an otherwise dull and dark time in my life.

Opening each package was fun. Many gifts made me cry, others helped me to laugh heartily, while some sent me into deep reflection.

The value of each gift was not the contents of the package but the time each dear sender had spent travelling to the shops, the time spent choosing the gift, the effort taken to wrap and package it and yet another journey to the post office to post it. When people give you of their valuable time, it's a treasured gift. You know they really care.

You may wonder what these packages contained:

Organic soaps and body care products, inspirational books and calendars, angel cards, candles, herbal teas, cancer books, audio books, funny DVD movies, meditation or restful music CD's, bandanas, symbolic trinkets, clothes, jewellery, a fleece blanket and pillow to take to chemo sessions, one friend sent her marathon medal (yes, can you believe it?), notebooks and pens for journaling and more.

Other gifts were hand-delivered:

Hands-on healing, hugs, cooked meals, soups, drives to hospitals and healers, visits, walking partners, companions to sit by my bed on the harder days, listening ears, moral support, shared information and experiences, help with house-work and the list goes on.

I would include cards, e-mails, text messages and letters in the gift category and there were endless numbers of each. No matter what was written on them, the message I understood loud and clear was "I care, you are not alone."

Don't underestimate the value of sending gifts, any gift. You can't even begin to imagine the support and love that comes attached.

You know for sure that there is someone out there somewhere that's thinking about you and sending love.

Most of all, keep in touch, no matter what.

GIFTS & WHAT THEY MEANT TO ME . . .

CONTACT

Contact during the cancer journey is the sun between the clouds, the energy that warms your heart and the assurance that you are not alone.

When 'sisters' text you day after day and month after month you know you are not alone. But, when people send extra special texts you cry just from the oneness of spirit. For example, the morning I was to have my head shaved a friend texted "Today is a different kind of pain . . ." She got it and she got it right. It was more than I needed that emotional morning. Once as I struggled through the early days post a chemo session I got a text that read "Today is day five . . ." Wow, it just blew me out of the water. This dear 'sister' had been texting me every day, I hadn't had the energy to reply, but she kept vigil with me anyway, counting the days, sticking with me no matter what.

Nieces and nephews sent cards and drawings that they had spent time decorating, to which they generously added their treasured stickers and pure wishes for my return to good health. From a child, it's so sweet, genuine and authentic—it really and truly heals.

Phone calls that started with "How are you?" and I was given time to reply meant everything. I so needed to share what was happening to me and for people to listen.

Visitors who came to help in a practical way, as opposed to just 'visit', were worth their weight in gold.

E-mails that showed caring, empathy, love and useful well-researched links, were so gratefully received.

Contact that didn't work for me was 'no contact', or contact that never included me at all—never referred to my condition, never enquired about my current state of health, never ended with even the simplest good wish for my recovery, test, surgery or whatever was current. Unfortunately, this kind of contact can push you into a state similar to grief. Fortunately for me, this kind of 'contact' was a rarity. I worked hard to vacate this thoughtless energy from my space, in order to leave even more room for all the wonderful, dear and generously considerate people who fortunately surrounded me for the entire duration of the journey.

THE KIND OF CONTACT I HAVE/NEED . . .

50

The idea of turning fifty had never been an issue for me. I had always been active (very!), energetic and enthusiastic about life. I poured my heart and soul into everything I did. I looked on the approaching new decade as just more of life to swallow whole. I'd imagined I'd wake up on the morning of my 50th birthday, throw my arms in the air and shout "I'm fifty and lovin' it." But . . . things didn't quite go according to plan!

Two days before my 50th birthday I'd received the 5th round of chemotherapy. By the time my birthday swung around, I was drowning in the full impact of the most challenging (understatement!) side-effects.

The fact that my Dad had died at age fifty and taking my own current situation into account changed how I woke up that morning. I now realized that reaching age fifty was a more significant achievement than I'd previously realized. I was lucky to be alive. As Jon Kabat Zinn wisely suggests—if you are breathing, your situation is a lot better than you realize!

So, as I opened my eyes on the morning of my 50th birthday and the full impact of pain and discomfort smacked me instantly, I still felt grateful. I was quite simply happy, relieved and thankful just to be alive. My head flooded with endless lists of reasons to be grateful and to enjoy this, yet another, wonderful day that lay ahead, no matter what physical shape I was in or what the day would bring. This day, and the joy of living it, as fully as I could under the circumstances, was my most precious birthday gift. I was humbled into a place of infinite gratitude and love for my life, as it was, on that day.

Did I register even a tiny note of disappointment, regret or upset at how my landmark birthday was playing out? No, not a trace! I knew just how fortunate I was to be alive at all and I just breathed into that.

I can't remember a day when I was so swamped in genuine love, compassion, caring and true empathy. An avalanche of cards, text messages, phone-calls, gifts, letters, e-mails, flowers, callers and kindness snowed me in and kept my rather frail body and fairly battered soul floating, smiling, serene, peaceful and quietly happy.

I cried at the end of my beautiful day. It had been more than perfect. This is how I would choose to live all my days from now on, seeing each day as the only day, the perfect and special day, the day to be grateful for, to live it fully and be 'in the moment', every moment of it.

Your cancer journey birthday is just another day, another beautiful pearl on the string of beads that is your life. Cherish it.

MY ___ CANCER JOURNEY
BIRTHDAY . . .

DOCTOR'S VISIT'S

Doctor's visits are a regular feature in my life now. I've grown accustomed to them. I no longer think about any discomfort that might be involved. I've been poked, prodded, injected, connected to machines, scanned and checked out so often that it no longer costs me a thought. I embrace every situation that I see as part of getting better or staying well.

A companion and a notebook are the two most important things you should bring to every doctor's visit. Sometimes you may feel too tired or unwell to concentrate enough to take in all the facts. When you have a companion with you the chance is higher that, between you, you will remember most, or all, of the information.

The day prior to your doctor's visit it's a great idea to write a list of questions to ask the doctor the next day. Sometimes we think we'll remember everything, but under the pressure of the moment, we often remember our most important questions after we have left the doctor's office! When you have your questions written in your notebook, ahead of time, this won't happen. The notebook also serves as the place to record important information the doctor tells you, for example, the dates of upcoming tests, or the date of your next appointment with him, or changes in the type of medication you need, or names of other specialists you may need to see. This special and important notebook also serves as a record for you of your progress. There is enormous satisfaction in seeing how well you are doing, especially when you work so hard on your wellness, daily. It feels good to be proactive in your own healing.

Your doctor is a human being just like you. You can feel relaxed with him, say how you feel, what you think and ask any question. You want information and you need feedback. Ask about every test, injection, scan, ultrasound and blood test before agreeing to it and ask to see the results too, when the time comes. When it comes to your body and your health, always ask. No question is too silly, too simple or too irrelevant to ask. Being proactive shows you are taking responsibility for your health and really want to recover. Even after major surgery, when I was completely 'out of it' I always opened one eye and, even with slurred speech, asked what was being injected into my IV.

If you still don't feel 100%, even if your doctor tells you that your test or scan was clear, persist and insist on further testing.

Your doctor will not be able to read your mind so you'll need to tell him how you feel, voice your fears and worries and say what you think, feel and need. You are in your own power when you speak and ask.

We now live in the age of information so of course we all google to find information about just about everything. Googling is very useful when you wish to familiarize yourself with hitherto unknown medical terms, or procedures and anything to do with your treatments that you don't understand. I feel some doctors are more comfortable with the expression "I was just wondering about . . ." as opposed to saying "I read on the internet!"

Ask your oncologist if there is anything you can do to help yourself. If he comes up with ideas— that's wonderful. If he says there isn't anything you can do at home between check-ups, then, think again! There is a whole world of things you can do to help keep yourself well. I think nutrition, exercise, rest, meditation, yoga, healing techniques of every kind, a positive attitude, affirmations, having fun and being in nature will go a long way towards 'you helping you'.

I feel it's of huge importance to express gratitude to doctors. They are our lifeline and tirelessly do everything they know how to do in order to cure us. A sincere thank you will go a long way. We all like to be thanked and appreciated from time to time and your doctor/oncologist needs that too.

DOCTOR'S VISITS . . .

WELLNESS

Wellness is always a choice, your choice. During the cancer/chemo journey I saw it as my life-line. In the early post treatments days I felt it was a life-sentence to always have to make the right choices about food, lifestyle and exercise. Now, I know for sure, that it's not a life-sentence but rather a way of life that keeps me healthy, well, able, strong, cheerful and alive. I know I have nothing to lose and everything to gain by adhering to my wellness programme.

When doing chemotherapy you can't take supplements, vitamins, herbal remedies, homeopathy or anything other than chemo itself. The chemo crushes your immune system to almost zero. You are weak, tired and ill. It feels at times as if you are barely hanging on to life by a thread. Your wellness choices are your only armor and defense against cancer and chemo. The return journey to good health and strength is a long haul. You have to earn your way. Sticking with your wellness programme keeps you strong.

I received chemotherapy and saw my oncologist every three weeks. Right from the start I felt three weeks was a long time between 'help'. I thought, I need to take responsibility for my own wellness and do everything in my power to enhance my own healing, between visits. It was clear that there was so much I could do to help and heal myself, and I did.

When I was sick, wellness took up most of my day because I was so tired, weak and moved so slowly. The simplest activity seemed to take forever. But, even on days when my energy level was in the minuses, my emotions were raw, I could barely walk or even keep my eyes open and pain was severe, I made the choice to be well and stuck with as many elements of my wellness programme as was physically possible for me, at that time.

Putting myself and my wellness first was a huge behavior change for me. Wellness was my work and it was a full-time job. There was no more important work for me at the time than getting well again. It was the main focus of my day, every day. I took doing everything I needed to do, to stay as well as I could, very seriously.

Wellness takes time, effort and energy. Don't say to yourself "I don't have time to walk," you do, you just choose to spend your time doing other things and you think you don't have time. I found time all day, every day, for about sixteen months, to be unwell!

When you are very ill you may have a great wellness programme but feel unable to implement it because you may not have enough energy or be too sick. You need people in your life, like never before—it really does 'take a village', till you are well enough again to do everything for yourself.

It can be very hard to find time for your wellness, to live mindfully, to take time to live as you feel you need to in order to stay healthy and well in mind, body and spirit. Life is life. You are either part of it or you are not. There are parts of everyday life that you can't run from, evade or ignore, for example, grocery shopping so you can maintain a healthy diet, taking care of your children, doctor's check-ups, alternative treatments, exercise, running your home, being part of a social network, celebrations of every kind, and more.

You may feel you don't have enough money to spend on organic food, alternative treatments or extra help of any kind, but you do, you just spend that money on other things—switch! Many of the most effective wellness ideas cost little or no money at all.

Do the important parts of your wellness programme while you feel well, possibly early in the morning, while you still have some energy. Even if you nap in the middle of the day, you may not have a lot of energy after that for the rest of the day.

Walk even if you feel tired. If you find it hard to get going alone, find someone to walk with you. It's the one sure way to get strong and stay strong.

My wellness programme changes from time to time but the basics stay the same. Let me share it with you.

Each of the following in the correct quantity, quality and frequency: water, food, rest, exercise and being in my own power. I also:

o Walk or go to the gym
o Make juice with fresh, organic fruit and vegetables
o Meditate/do Reiki
o Do breathing exercises
o Say affirmations
o Eat a healthy, fresh, organic diet
o Take a nap (at least twenty minutes)
o Get seven hours sleep at night
o Do something that's fun, for me
o Connect with loved ones
o Get out in nature
o Read
o Try to make a difference in the world.

The power to create what we think and believe to be true lies within each one of us. Decide what wellness means for you and go for it. It's as simple as that. Don't give up just because you think it's disguised as hard work—it's not disguised, it actually **is** hard work!

People who have never done a cancer journey can be casual, or even lazy, about their wellness. They put off the work of wellness, promising that they will get around to it later, but may never. A Champ could never allow herself the luxury of such a risk, the stakes are too high.

I'll most likely stick with my wellness programme for the rest of my life. I feel so well living like this that I wouldn't ever want to live differently again. I know that good health does not happen by chance, I need to work at it. Wellness is no longer a chore but a choice. I no longer adhere to my wellness programme out of fear of being sick, but rather, I do it for the joy of feeling well. Today I am well and I'm prepared to do whatever it takes so ensure that I stay that way.

MY WELLNESS
PROGRAMME . . .

DEPRESSION

That dreaded word, depression. Yes, it's definitely part of the cancer journey at one time or another. For some it's something that comes, stays a while and disappears. There are other people for whom it comes, sticks and they just can't seem to shake it off.

Depression on a cancer journey is unlike depression at other times in life, in that, the causes, duration and cures may be different.

There are Champs who are on their first 'round of the track' with cancer and can feel depressed because:

o They are sick
o Their 'old' life is over
o They can't participate fully in 'real' life
o They feel that the journey is endless
o They can't see any light at the end of the tunnel
o They may feel that life will never be the same again for them afterwards
o No one really understands what they feel or fear
o They fail to function 'normally'.

Some Champs are on their second or third 'trip' with cancer and so for them depression can be the result of:

o   Over-exposure to pain
o   Treatment's harsh side-effects
o   Aloneness
o   Fear of not making it
o   Sadness that they can't be there for their families in the capacity that they would wish
o   Regrets
o   Raw feelings regarding physical changes and body malfunctions
o   Disbelief about lack of expected support and such like.

Depression can set in when you least expect it. You can feel in good form one morning and by noon your heart is in your shoes. In some cases it can help to ask "Why am I depressed?" because once you know, you can do something to change the events that caused you to feel this way. At other times it can be easier to just let go of those depressed feelings without analyzing why you feel like that—just hand it over and let it go. If depression sets in and doesn't go away after three weeks or so, it's best to seek professional help—that could take the form of counseling, medication or whatever else the doctor orders.

Personally, although I generally have a 'sunny' nature, I experienced depression from time to time throughout the cancer journey. The duration of each bout varied from hours, to a couple of days. The longest session, which was three weeks, was a very deep, dark, bleak, black hole. It was with the greatest difficulty that I climbed my way back to the light from there.

Here are a few helpful hints on how to help yourself stay depression-free and how to stop yourself falling further, if you should sense yourself slipping in that direction:

o Meditation
o Listen to any music, that for you, is restful
o Get out in fresh air, no matter what the season—if it's raining just go anyway with an umbrella
o Exercise—you may not be able for more than a short, slow walk, but move in whatever way and to whatever capacity you are capable of, at this time
o Make sure you get enough rest—sometimes depression (on the cancer journey) can set in when we feel physically overwhelmed or exhausted and getting enough rest can curtail that
o Avoid contact with people that upset you, don't resonate with you or are in any way 'toxic' for you at this challenging time
o Get into gratitude mode or develop a better gratitude attitude—once you start thinking of things to be grateful for the whole picture can change for you
o Become more aware of all the love, compassion, kindness, thoughtfulness and

generosity of spirit around you—let that light seep into your being and your broken spirit

o Try to do something small for someone else, even the smallest gesture will do—call and ask how someone else is doing, thank a friend who is doing so much to help you, support another Champ, hug your children or do anything that involves reaching out past yourself to another sweet soul

o Remind yourself that if you allow yourself to fall further than you already have that the climb back to feeling good will take longer and be even more complicated and challenging

o Take your time, don't stress or rush, be gentle with yourself. Sometimes when we feel depressed on this journey it's just part of it and if we flow with it for a day or two someone's thoughtful behavior, a loving gesture, a kind act, a gift in the post, a sign from the Universe, good energy coming your way, a smiling visitor, a passage you read in an inspirational book, a sudden change for the better (even slightly) in your physical well-being, or good news from your oncologist might just be the catalyst that will swing your mood and depressed feelings around to a more positive direction.

Every part of the cancer journey is different for everyone—how the symptoms present themselves, how your body reacts to chemotherapy, and even how quickly your body heals after surgery. It's also different for you how often you'll feel low or depressed, for how long you may feel like that and how quickly you'll succeed in pulling yourself back to a safe, centered and grounded position again.

WHEN I'M DEPRESSED . . .

WHAT NOT TO DO OR SAY!

It's completely understandable that there are people who have never experienced cancer on any level. Dealing with your cancer may be a first for them. We need to be patient and accept the fact that sometimes people just don't know what to do or say—it's all new to them.

Here are a few tips on what **not** to do or say:

Don't take photos of a champ without asking first. I remember, during the early days of my journey, a friend came to visit. When I saw her remove her camera from her bag my heart missed a beat. I thought, oh no, she thinks I'm not going to make it and wants to have a souvenir photo! In fact, the truth was that she wanted to show me some shots she'd taken the previous day! Just think about how adults fuss before being photographed when they are healthy and well. Try to envision how hard it may be for some Champs to have their photograph taken, when they may be looking and feeling the worst they ever have in their lives.

Don't keep talking to a Champ about someone else you know who has done a cancer journey, how well they coped with their treatments, how they worked through it all or how fast they recovered. It may give the Champ the idea that they are not measuring up, not coping as well as others do or not being enough. Just listen to the Champ that's in your presence now. This journey is so challenging that comparisons don't have a place.

When you call and ask a Champ how they are, they will tell you. Give them time to explain how there are doing, they have earned that.

Don't send anything to a Champ, who is still doing their journey, about another Champ who has died. You may argue that it's part of the reality of cancer, life and the real world. There is a time and a place for everything in life and this is not the time for a Champ to hear about a fellow traveller of the cancer journey who didn't make it. All Champs are acutely aware that not every Champ makes it, but one doesn't need reminding! Try to imagine if you were a Champ how you'd feel on receiving such news.

You don't need to ask a Champ to support cancer causes. She already has/is! She has already done the journey and in so doing has supported the cause. Every woman who has done the journey has been an involuntary victim of research, science, medicine, cures and treatments to move forward in unimaginable ways. A Champ will also be able to support another Champ in ways that no one else ever will—because she really knows, understands and 'gets' it. If she wants to give further support she'll come to it herself. It's hard to imagine what seeing the word 'cancer' triggers in a cancer survivor—so use the word sparingly in the company (mails, texts, calls and visits) of a Champ.

It can be annoying when people who haven't been with you on the journey start telling you what you do, what you should be doing and what you shouldn't be doing. Sometimes it's people who live far away and are not part of your day to day life, who have no way at all of knowing how you live your life on a day to day basis, who make the most bizarre suggestions. They may think they know what you're doing but they can't possibly. Their knowledge of what they think you are doing is based solely on the person you were pre-cancer. Well, that person has long since vanished and disappeared, she no longer exists. You are different now. You think differently, feel differently, see life differently and behave differently. Believe me, a Champ really knows what she should or shouldn't be doing . . . and how!

When a Champ tells you she is afraid, don't tell her she doesn't need to be—she already **is** afraid! Her fear is real, natural and needs to be felt—you only need to listen. Maybe instead of telling her not to be afraid you could ask her what her biggest fear is and just listen.

Don't start any form of communication, with a Champ, with anything other than "How are you?" Don't forget to wait for the answer! That little question can change everything for a Champ.

Don't ask a Champ "What else are you doing?" when they have told you about their chemo, pain, surgery or challenging time. When you are doing chemo, that's all there is, there just isn't room in your life for anything else—as it is, you can barely cope with just that.

Don't have **any** expectations of a Champ while on her cancer journey. You can't have even the vaguest notion of how challenging this journey is unless you have experienced it personally . . . and may you never!

Don't compare cancer patients who have different cancers or even cancer patients who have the same type of cancer. Even patients with the same type of cancer, receiving the same type of treatment and drugs may feel and react differently. Everyone and everyone's body reacts in an individual way.

When a Champ has waited day after endless day for test results, a call from her oncologist, news of the date for an upcoming treatment or surgery, please don't tell her how absurd, ridiculous or outrageous the medical system is that she has been kept waiting for so long. Who knows better than the Champ how long the wait has been? Who is more anxious than the Champ to get answers? Do you really think it encourages calm, inspires confidence in the system and is helpful to the Champ when you verbally shred the medical system that she's dependent on to save her life? No! Please, please, please, choose instead to ask if the Champ would like some company or to go out for a coffee. Re-assure the Champ that it can't be long more now till she gets her answer. Remind the Champ that you are with her in spirit, here if she needs you and that you feel sure all is well. You'll know how best to handle it if you imagine yourself to be in the Champ's place. How would you like the conversation to go? What words of encouragement would you like to hear as you wait, wait and wait some more? Also think about words you definitely wouldn't need to hear as you sit in a state of high anxiety, watching your clock! Think, feel, listen and then speak.

Never drop by a Champ's home without calling first. You can't know what state or condition the Champ is in that day, at that moment. She may be unable to get out of bed, she may feel low and unlike socializing, she may not be dressed, she may be asleep, she may be in too much pain to cope with a visitor or any myriad of genuine reasons why it's better to call first if you plan on visiting a Champ, any time, any day, always.

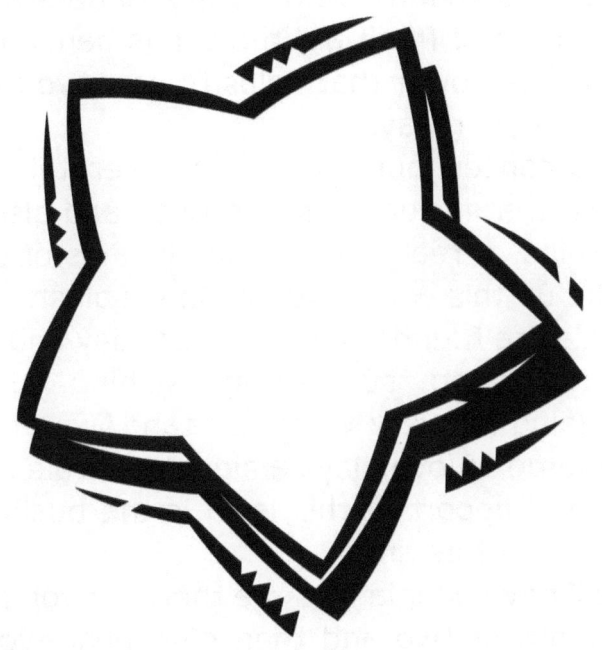

The light of a star is only visible in juxtaposition to the darkness that surrounds it.

IT TAKES ALL KINDS

The relationships in our lives play a central role in how we cope with illness, especially this illness. Talking to someone who **really** understands is like a breath of fresh air, the wings beneath your feet and the power that helps to carry you a little further on your way.

On a cancer journey you see everything as it really is, that includes life, yourself and also your friendships. It really does take all kinds of people to make up this wonderful world we all share!

There are friends who are there day and night, listening, caring, supporting, wishing you well and helping in every way they can. Awareness of that volume of love plays a significant role in your recovery. Support at this level is the business of friendship at this time.

You'll have people who are there for you for the first month or two and then disappear—you can deal with that because it's in those first months when life is most challenging for you, when you're getting used to so many changes and letting go of your old life. You may feel fearful, physically weak and the road ahead may look so long as it stretches out in front of you. This is a time when you can use all the support you can get. Later, when you are more established in your situation (hard as it may be) you can manage with smaller numbers of constant companions.

There are others who know you are ill (you may have told them yourself!) and yet, when they meet you they never make any reference to it, or enquire about your current state of health. Those of you doing the journey, will have had phone calls from time to time, from people who talk endlessly about everything that is going on in their own lives and never stop, for a second, to simply ask "How are you?" . . . not forgetting the all important second step . . . to wait for your reply! Who knows, maybe it's just all too hard for them, maybe they are fearful of being ill themselves one day, maybe a loved one has died of the illness you now have or maybe they just don't know what to say. Focus on the people who are supportive, helpful and loyal. Let go, without judgment, of the one or two who can't handle your situation.

There is yet another category of friend—the friend who cares, is interested and keeps in touch but you, on the other hand, do not feel connected to her, at this time. It doesn't mean that the friend is getting it wrong. It just means that you can't connect with her, but you do appreciate the show of concern and interest, even if you are not on the same wavelength, for the moment.

There are a few who can't even say the word 'cancer' or can't bear to be with someone who is doing the journey. For reasons of their own, they need to get far away from anything to do with it. I'd put it down to fear or past experience of their own. The thing to do is to just accept the situation as it is and let go.

It's hard, next to impossible in fact, to go it alone on this path. It's a time of huge anxiety for the Champ, all day, every day, until it's over.

If you have spare energy (!), sit quietly and make a list of the people in your life. Take a moment to ponder which relationships nourish your soul, which ones you need to put on hold and which ones are downright toxic, no longer resonate with you and you must extricate yourself from immediately. This exercise is not about blame but about suitability—it's a 'yes/no' question:

o Does this relationship work for me now?

o Does this person make me feel peaceful, joyful, serene and relaxed or do I feel upset, tense, tearful, triggered and low after spending time with them?

It only takes a second to figure it out, because your heart already knows the answer. Treasure the friendships that nurture you and let go of any relationship that, for you, is toxic.

So, there are those who are indescribably loyal and get it right and there are those for whom it's too hot in the kitchen, so they have to get out. Even though you are deeply hurt at being abandoned, try not to judge them, just let them go with love and gratitude.

Remember that when someone leaves your circle, it leaves room for someone new to enter.

Love and listening are the most needed friendship qualities for a Champ on a cancer journey. Those beautiful, special and faithful friends who accompany you make up for any friend who drops out. Forgive and let go, with a heart filled with love and a soul packed with gratitude, that you are blessed beyond measure to be able to count such dear people on even one hand.

UNTANGLING THE 'SALAD' IN MY HEAD . . .

A JOURNEY ENDS

When you meet a friend through cancer, it's a friendship with a difference, from day one. You bypass the looking good/feeling good stage and there is never anything superficial about any element of it, ever.

When Edie crossed paths with me, I was bald and she'd already had cancer twice!

From the start we tuned in to one another. There was perfect understanding, acceptance and empathy. Explanations of any kind were unnecessary.

Edie was ahead of me in 'the game'. She warmly, patiently and lovingly guided me. She understood what it meant and how I was feeling if mails, text messages or calls went unanswered for days. She knew when I needed cheering on or cheering up. She understood when I needed space and withdrew . . . but she was still there, waiting, watching and wishing me well. It was an easy, comfortable friendship because it never required explanations, apologies or excuses. It was completely stress free and in the moment. It just was as it was.

I'd already finished my treatments when a tumour was discovered in Edie's brain. It meant cancer number three for her and more surgery. I was astounded by the grace and acceptance with which she approached her ordeal. She was so positive.

She picked up incredibly well after her surgery. Then, within weeks she fell into a 'big, black hole'. It took her weeks to crawl out, but she did.

She was doing so well. She'd learned so much. She'd internalized so many universal principles and made them her own. She saw life as it really was.

The final blow came when cancer invaded her pancreas. She accepted it with peace. It seemed to me that she expected to recover and get well again.

I visited her at home, about three weeks before her journey ended. She was dressed and wearing make-up. We sat in the shade of a huge protective tree in her garden. The energy there was magical. We sat in harmony of soul, drinking water and sharing lessons learned. At this stage Edie radiated tranquility, serenity and calm. It was infectious.

Words were unnecessary. We were on the same page. We comfortably rode silence.

We accepted our situations as they were. We didn't waste a moment griping, complaining, moaning, crying, fussing or wondering 'why me?' We didn't blame. We were living in the moment.

We were grateful to have this special time together, to share and be in the safe embrace of the tree in her garden. It didn't matter what tomorrow would bring.

When I left Edie that day I had no idea that I'd never see her again. She never gave any indication that she might not make it. She spoke like someone who was fully alive and in love with life.

On hearing that Edie had passed away tears flooded my being. I cried out of sadness that this beautiful woman, this special soul that had shared my journey at such a critical time, no longer breathed life. Her journey had ended. She was at peace now. She was on the vacation she'd spoken so often about taking "When this is all over."

I didn't at any point feel that her journey was my journey. I knew our destinies were separate. It was clear to me that Edie's time had come. It was the end of her journey but not necessarily mine, right now.

I feel enormous gratitude to Edie for everything we shared. She touched my life in a very real way from the start. She has left me with huge awareness and understanding. I remember her wise words in phone-calls, her cheery supportive text messages, her always appropriate and in-tune mails.

Knowing Edie has been an honour of the highest order. Letting go feels like an open wound. Celebrating all that she meant to me is a privilege. May you rest in peace, Edie.

I want to share with you a beautiful and exceedingly special piece that Edie sent me after she was cured of cancer for the second time. I see it as her legacy to the world.

The Sun Shines Beyond the Clouds

The sun **always shines** beyond the clouds. The cloud of cancer that hung over me for four years lifted and my heart is shining again. Please God, it's behind me forever. Yahoo . . . Yippee! I celebrate my health and wellness. Throughout this roller coaster journey, I viewed myself as healthy, while my body was fighting cancer. I've learned so much. The biggest lesson—we are so much more than our physical being.

In December 2004 I was diagnosed with bladder cancer. "It's slow-growing, non-aggressive and you can live with it for thirty years," said my urologist. I took it as a challenge to face my fears and pave a path to wellness. After five surgeries and two rounds of treatments, cancer has not grown in my bladder in more than a year! However, last February, they found cancer on my lung. Do you believe it? I'm a nice girl from Ohio that never smoked. As we all know, life's full of surprises. So, during chemo, which I renamed silver rain, I enjoyed long visits with Mordechai and friends. It shrank by 50% (I had hoped for a disappearing act). I gave myself two days to adjust to the new reality of surgery. My surgeon told me he had patients who ran marathons after this surgery. Maybe now I'll run a marathon I thought! Five days after surgery I was home and working towards my coaching certification, a goal I've had for a long time. I continued to stay focused on goals and where I was headed!

Three months after surgery, Mordechai and I walked up five hundred and thirty five steps to see an amazing waterfall in Sloveania. I'm filled with infinite love and gratitude for all those who were with me through this. First my family . . . I love you with all my heart. So many friends called, sent emails, cards, food, visits and loving energy. I am grateful to the professionals who helped me align my body and mind. My medical doctors gave me opportunity to trust their expertise while I learned to listen to my intuition. A wide variety of complimentary professionals believed in me often more than I believed in myself, particularly Dr. Roy Gonik, who practices an amazing technique called LIFE LINE, which taps into our body's wisdom. I learned from healer Maurice to focus on what I want in life, not my fears. I'm eternally grateful for my deepened trust in God, who guided me to my strength, courage, wisdom and inner peace.

I want to share with you a few lessons I've learned:

- o Focus on what you want (for me it was health vs. the absence of cancer)
- o Trust your intuition
- o Find the bright side
- o Have courage to face darkness
- o Believe after darkness there is light
- o Let others be there for you

o   Ask for what **you** want!
o   Choose to host thoughts that lift you
o   Accept others
o   Be grateful
o   Cry when you feel the urge
o   Laugh even when you do not feel the urge
o   Breathe, breathe, breathe . . . your life
    depends on it!

I chose to breathe fully into my life and live as if I am cured forever! I will not let today pass me by because I'm afraid what might happen. This is what I wish for you too!

Edie Ilan (December, 2008)

LOSING A FRIEND TO CANCER . . .

READ & KNOW

Knowledge is power. There has never been a time in your life when this statement holds more substance than on your cancer journey. Ignorance is not bliss at this time!

What should you read? Reading about your own type of cancer is a great place to start. You could read on the internet or relevant books. Survivor's stories are a great source of information, validation and comfort because you read about real people who have already completed the journey you are now on. It gives you hope knowing that if they did it that you can too.

There are people who fear reading the facts and statistics of what may lie ahead for them. In particular they may have worries about reading on the internet, because they may read information there that could worry them. I believe that nothing beats doing some research and being prepared for your doctor's visits, scans, procedures, tests, treatments and the journey ahead. The unknown is infinitely more terrifying than the truth, even if the truth is unpleasant.

Once you know what may lie ahead, you can take more responsibility for your health, your recovery and your wellness. When you can see the path ahead and the target, you know where you are going and what you have to do to get there.

As a result, instead of being a passive patient, you can be an important participant of your own medical team and an active patient in your own healing and recovery.

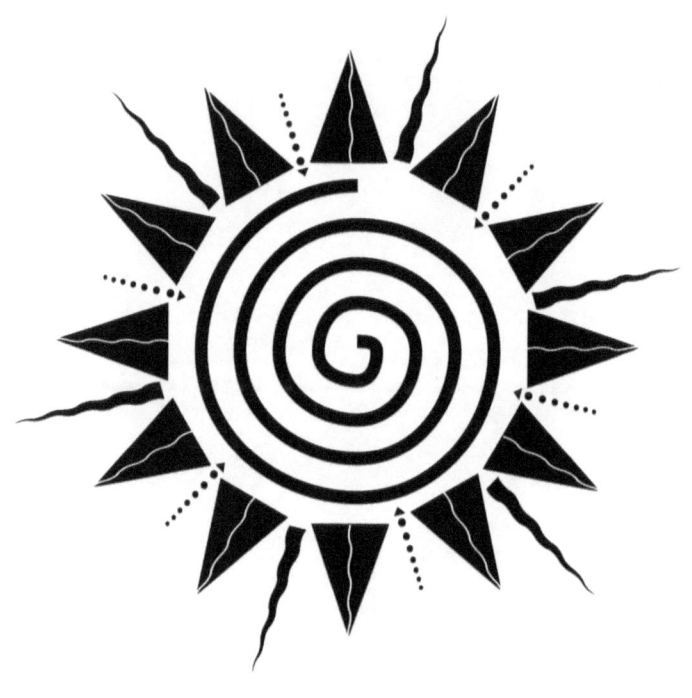

Radiating optimistically out from the
centre,
Full of endless possibilities,
It speaks of a journey from past to
future.

BEST BOOKS

We all know that knowledge is power. At no other time, more than when doing a cancer journey, do we need to be informed. The problem is, that although we are most likely off work and not doing all the running around that we usually engage in, we don't read that much. We plan on reading, we wish to read but it doesn't happen simply because we have neither the focus nor the energy for it, at this time.

With this in mind I want to share with you the names of the few books that, for me, were easiest to read, the most helpful and held the seeds of wisdom I actually needed to hear at the time. I was able to readily incorporate the ideas into my everyday life without too much fuss or effort. Most of what we need to know about our chemotherapy drugs/treatment, our scans, tests and surgeries can be read about on the internet.

These books give you what you won't find on the internet and are all written by cancer survivors, which of course is key; they know, understand and appreciate every element of what you are going through. It might be a good idea to read them in the order listed.

- o THE CHOICE by Bernadette Bohan
- o THE JOURNEY by Brandon Bays
- o SURVIVING CANCER edited by Paul Kraus

THE CHOICE is a book everyone should read, not just someone on a cancer journey. Bernadette survived cancer twice. In her book she shares an easy to read, follow and implement four-step plan that helped save her own life—juicing, power foods, pure water and safe toiletries. She shows how little it takes to make a huge difference to your health. Bernadette explains simply and clearly the 'why' and 'how to' of the juices, food, safe water and toiletries. This must-have book also includes recipes, the type you really could and would adopt and make part of your everyday life.

THE JOURNEY is just that, the story of Brandon's own journey through cancer and out the other side to perfect health and a vibrant life. Brandon actually stumbled on a healing method as she worked on her own wellness, which she called 'The Journey'. I loved her book. It was a light but very moving, informative and 'real' read. When I completed my own treatments I did a three-day workshop with Brandon Bays, did some treatments, learned about The Journey technique myself and how to apply it. The book gives great insight into how important a part we play in our own healing and how our bodies are perfect healing organisms.

SURVIVING CANCER is a collection of short stories written by long-term survivors. The time to read this book is when you have finished your treatments, but before you feel really healthy and 'normal' again. The stories are written by cancer survivors who survived multiple 'tours' with cancer.

By the time I'd read the last story some common denominators had surfaced. It was clear that long term survivors:

o Take their wellness seriously, every single day
o Understand that wellness is the most important element of their day
o Exercise, meditate, juice, eat a vegetarian diet
o Make lots of changes in their lives
o Learn to live in the moment
o Experience huge gratitude
o Want to share what they have learned and help others on their cancer journeys
o Place huge value on alternative treatments, alongside conventional cures
o Have a positive outlook on life
o Never give up hope

There are endless cancer books on the market but these three, for me, were superior, in that, they really shared what I needed to hear, learn and apply. I could easily relate to them. They were written by real people who had actually done the journey and knew exactly what they were talking about, what worked and what didn't work, what changes one needs to make and the help that is available.

WISE & MEANINGFUL BOOKS . . .

CARERS

The cancer journey is a bit like a storm at sea, it requires 'all hands on deck' for survival. When you do a cancer journey, everyone who lives at your home does the journey with you. Everyone's life is affected, changes and evolves with yours, each in his own way and at his own pace.

How could one possibly make it on this journey alone? I dread to think where we would be without our loyal, loving, devoted and tirelessly giving carers who look after our every need when we can do little more than just perform the most basic functions alone. Their support in our healing, their belief that we will make it, their help and love should never be under-estimated, or taken for granted.

Who are these carers? Carers are the people (if you are fortunate enough to have them in your life!) who take care of everything that you are too unwell to do for yourself, while you are ill. You may think that the list would include going to the supermarket, preparing dinner and walking your dog—and you'd be right. But there is so much more to it than that.

There are days when you are so bewildered, dazed and lost that their caring, compassion, love and kindness are all you have to hold on to and give you the drive to carry on for another day.

Carers are the ones who understand and comfort you when you are crying and you don't even know why yourself. On days when you are unable to drive, they drive you to healers, doctor's appointments and everywhere else you need to go. They prepare food to nourish your frail body and make vegetable juices to fill you with antioxidants, vitamins and minerals. Even on days when they don't feel a bit like walking, they will walk with you to keep you strong and hold you up, when you can't even climb onto the footpath by yourself. They make sure there is food on the table for your children while you take the nap you need, but they can't allow themselves the luxury of a nap right now. Carers listen. Carers are generous with hugs when they realize that there are no appropriate words to 'fix' things. Carers are compassionate when you can barely get out of bed, function, contribute to family life, perform even the simplest tasks or be sociable.

You will be grateful to note that they are with you when you start your journey and are still loyally and faithfully there six months later at the end of your treatments and surgeries. Needless to add, they will still be by your side yet a year later when you have finally recovered and healed.

Carers are often forgotten in everyone's anxiety about the cancer patient. We need to remember that carers juggle their lives on a daily basis and take on your role as well as living their own. Without warning they suddenly have lots of choices removed from the 'menu' of their own lives as they become flexible and on call 24/7. Your health may have been temporarily taken away but the carers time, freedom of choice, fun, schedule, relaxation time and whole life has also been turned upside-down too. We need to remember that, with love and gratitude, at all times.

For me, it was a stunning realization that I was so deeply loved. I'd spent my entire life giving and loving to such an extent that I was completely unaware of all the love and support that was coming my way.

I feel the need to endlessly and eternally praise the endurance of those who loved and cared for me at a time in my life when all I could do, at times, was just sit and breathe. As Elizabeth Gilbert says "Maybe it's wiser to surrender before the miraculous scope of human generosity and to just keep saying thank you, forever and sincerely, for as long as we have voices."

P.S. Now is the opportunity to learn to receive, if you are someone who has difficulty asking for and accepting help. Make it easier for your kind, considerate, compassionate and helpful carers by being specific about the kind of help you need—they genuinely want to help and they need to know how.

BLESS THEIR BEAUTIFUL & UNCONDITIONALLY LOVING HEARTS . . .

STUFF YOU SHOULD KNOW

There are many myths and popularly held beliefs, about various elements of the cancer journey, which are inaccurate. Let's mash some myths!

I'm 'doing nothing':

When a Champ says she is 'doing nothing', that is exactly what she means. She doesn't mean that she is relaxing with a good book, watching a funny movie, chatting with a friend on the phone or catching up on stuff at home. What a Champ means by 'doing nothing' is that she is most likely lying in bed, not moving, looking at the ceiling! That is all she is capable of, at that moment in time, and it can go on for hours or all day.

I'm 'not able':

If a Champ tells you she's not able to do something, she means just that. No matter how you word your suggestion, no matter what change you make to the basic plan, no matter who else might be involved, no matter how long or short the duration of the activity, 'not able' means just that. It means that the Champ is unable for any form of, or any element of, whatever you are suggesting, at this time.

I feel 'well':

When a Champ says she feels well she doesn't mean she feels well like you do, you are healthy. What she most likely means by 'well' is, that relative to yesterday, or earlier today, or relative to all that she has going on, that at this moment she feels relatively well—she doesn't know how long feeling 'well' will last, it can change at any moment.

I'm fearful:

When a Champ who has finished treatments talks about being fearful, she is most likely not talking about fear of death—which is what you may think she is afraid of. No, she is most likely fearful of cancer recurring. There is nothing more dreaded, or terrifying, in the mind of a Champ, than the idea of being sick again. Death may even come in second place for most Champs.

Pain killers kill pain:

Pain killers don't necessarily kill all pain. They may ease the pain, dull the pain or take the edge off it, but pain can still be felt—lots of pain, at times.

Nausea and vomiting:

Everyone doing chemotherapy has nausea and vomiting. No, not true. The side-effects of chemo depend on the combination of drugs given and also depend on the individual. Two patients can be given the same drugs and each may react differently. Each case is different.

When someone is going to die:

The doctor can know when someone is going to die. No, he can't. We all know that only one 'person' knows that—and it's not the doctor!

It's like the flu or being pregnant:

Sometimes when you tell someone about your side effects they'll chirp in that it's the same as having the flu or being pregnant! Having had the flu, been pregnant and done chemotherapy I can assure you that chemotherapy's side-effects are not like anything else, they are in a league of their own, they cannot be compared to anything else.

NOT AFRAID

I've lost count of the number of people who, at various stages of the journey, have asked me "Are you afraid?" My answer is always the same, "No." Needless to add, this draws comments as to how strong and brave I am! My answer is the truthful answer, to the question asked, but in answering honestly I've come to realize that I'm leading the questioner astray!

I've learned to let go of outcomes so I live in an open-ended way. I don't see ahead of time what the end of anything is. I can't know whether I'll be sick again, for how long I'll be well, what my quality of life will be, or answers about any element of my life. So, I live **d**efinitely **d**etached from **o**bsession **o**ver **o**utcomes (ddooo)! In this way I can, without fail, embrace life to the full.

When someone tells you they are not afraid, please don't misinterpret that. Don't equate lack of fear with lack of emotion. Even with a smile on one's face and a brave heart, it can be raining torrentially in one's already flooded soul.

Interestingly, the fear question is the one I'm always asked and no one, and I mean not even one person, has ever asked me whether I'm sad or not. Now, to this question I can answer a resounding **YES**! I feel sure I can speak for a large percentage of Champs when I say that, at times, we are lost and drowning in sadness.

This sadness isn't connected with death, feeling that you won't make is, lack of hope or negative thinking. No, it's just pure, undiluted, genuine emotion. It's about feeling all your feelings.

Sadness, for Champs, is generally not about past events, (I'd see those as regrets), or disappointment (that would be current) but rather about the possible loss of future experiences that may never be theirs to enjoy. Like what? Well:

o The possibility of not living to be older, the sense of something being snatched away and cut short

o The idea that you may not be around to applaud your children's future achievements

o The prospect, perhaps, of not being there to see your children wed

o The notion that you may never cuddle your first grandchild in your arms, or enjoy hearing yourself called Grandma

o The grief of maybe not being here to advise, help, support and guide your children

o The tragedy of possibly never happily sharing future good times, special occasions or golden moments with your family

o The trauma of knowing that you may not be available when things fall apart for your adult children, when life teaches them something the hard way, when they need to revert to being a kid for a bit and you may be absent o Missing out on later stages in life with your partner, 'sisters' and loved ones

o The heart-break of knowing that, if you don't make it, you'll break your loved one's hearts, steep them in grief and, as a direct result, change the course of their lives, from 'whenever' day forth.

At the most unexpected times, people, movies and events can trigger tears and an overwhelming sense of loss. It all comes under the umbrella of sadness.

So, if you know a champ who appears to be strong, brave, upbeat, calm and 'together' as she crawls on her journey, that's just her way of dealing, in a dignified way, with a challenge, that should she give it free rein may engulf, swamp and drown her within seconds.

MY GREATEST FEARS . . .

MY DEEPEST SADNESS . . .

THE UNIVERSE

"When a person really desires something, the Universe conspires to help that person to realize his dream," Paulo Coelho.

You may think you are a complete unit, separate and not connected to anything or anyone else, but you are part of the Universe. You are part of the whole. Everything you think, say and do affects you and everyone else. Early on my journey I became aware of that special connection. I could see that so many others were learning along-side me, were making changes in line with what was happening to me and were moving forward in different directions as a result of how they observed my life evolving.

You operate in harmony with the Universe. When you change your thoughts, words or attitude in life, the Universe mirrors that and sends you back more of the same. You reap what you sow, that's how the law of the Universe works. When I opened my heart to the Universe I noticed that magical things began to happen in my life. I didn't feel alone. I knew that I was being helped. I knew deep within my heart that no matter how challenging the journey became that I'd be given the tools, strength and guidance to cope. And so it was.

There has never been a time in my life when I needed help more than I did on the cancer journey. At this time I needed to ask for the help I needed, trust, let go and believe with all my heart that the Universe would provide. It did and how.

The Universe provided everything I needed on the cancer journey. I didn't fuss or worry, I just asked and waited. I trusted, with every fibre of my being, that all would be well. Everything I needed arrived at my feet. I was deeply moved. Every time things worked out perfectly, I just smiled a special smile that I reserve only for recognition of and gratitude to the Universe. It's a smile that says, "I know you are here with me, I don't feel alone, I trust you, I'm grateful."

Let me give you an idea of what I'm talking about:

I am truly blessed to be part of a wonderful, caring, endlessly loving and supportive family.

Just days before the cancer journey began, my daughter started at a new school where she was very happy, which brought me great joy.

My son had just finished high-school and was at home for the first months of treatments. He couldn't possibly have done more to help.

My brother-in-law, a talented chef, kindly came to cook many times, often after his twelve hour shifts at work. He cheerfully cooked all the healthy foods I required at this time.

A dear friend drove me to Dorit, my healer friend, a few days after each chemo session, once I could manage the journey but was still unable to drive myself.

I still had two more chemo sessions to complete and my son was no longer free to be at home, but the Universe came up trumps again. For each of my last chemo sessions a sister flew in from overseas to be with me during the first challenging week post each chemo session.

When I wasn't well enough to travel, healer friends offered to do healing sessions for me, in my own home.

Friends and extended family cooked for my family for more than six months.

Friends and loved ones sent packages in the post always containing the right inspirational material, comforting gift or treat.

I seemed to find myself in the hands of the right doctors, oncologists, professors and in the best hospital and chemo unit.

Friends flew in from overseas with the sole purpose of supporting me during chemotherapy or surgery.

Doctor's appointments, scans, ultrasounds, chemo sessions and so forth all, without exception, fitted in perfectly around my daughter's school schedule.

Cards, e-mails, text-messages, phone-calls, letters and visitors always seemed to arrive at exactly the time when I felt most vulnerable and in need of reassurance, contact, love and support.

I have always been a great believer in the power of the Universe, in the way it operates and in the abundance of the 'like attracting like' phenomenon.

There are no mistakes, chance occurrences or coincidences in the Universe. Everything happens at exactly the right time, in the right way and in the right order. I like to call this Divine Order. My requests and prayers were always heard. I didn't always get what I 'wanted' but I definitely got what I 'needed'.

When you consider that there are billions of people in the world, each and every one of them with their own problems and issues, it amazes me to think of the Universe finding space to pay attention to my every need. I know for sure that, in the Universe, all is exactly as it's meant to be at any given time, and as a result, all is well in my world—even if I'm doing a cancer journey, having multiple surgeries, wading my way through challenging treatments, struggling with recovery, or feeling uncertain. There is deep comfort in believing in the calm, strength and abundance of the Universe, 24/7.

I ASK, LET GO, TRUST
AND WAIT . . .

SIGNS AND SYMPTOMS

I'm sure you've heard Ovarian Cancer described as 'the silent killer'. You may have probed deeper and questioned the exact meaning of this. You were most likely told that "There are no signs or symptoms, so usually, by the time ovarian cancer is discovered, it's already too late." Sound familiar? If you've carried this myth around till now, let me inform you that it's not quite true! Ovarian cancer may be a killer but it's not silent—yes, there **are** signs and symptoms!

There are signs and symptoms but they are often missed, not so much by the woman who feels them, but by the doctor she goes to in search of an explanation as to why she feels like this. Some doctors are just not familiar enough with ovarian cancer to suspect that your symptoms may indeed be connected with a killer disease.

Looking at the symptoms, you can see why these apparently common, but slightly vague symptoms, could be so easily missed or misdiagnosed:

o Abdominal fullness or bloating
o Urinary urgency
o Pelvic discomfort or pain
o Persistent indigestion, gas or nausea
o Unexplained changes in bowel habits, e.g. constipation
o A frequent need to urinate

o Loss of appetite or feeling full quickly
o Pain during intercourse
o A persistent lack of energy
o Lower back pain
o Changes in menstruation

In fairness, some of the above symptoms could be attributed to a tired, overstressed, and possibly menopausal woman. One could understand how such symptoms may not seem serious, but they need to be taken seriously, because they could be early warning signs of ovarian cancer. Just because many of the symptoms are similar to other common complaints does not excuse any doctor who may bother a woman off again and again. Missing the correct diagnosis is unforgivable—just because the apparently simple symptoms can be easily explained away, does not mean that they will just go away.

As women, we need to educate ourselves about the symptoms of ovarian cancer. If you have already been diagnosed with any of the above symptoms and the prescribed treatment does not bring you relief after a few weeks, then schedule a return visit to your doctor, or get a second opinion. It could save your life!

Facts you should know:

o Ovarian cancer is the deadliest of all the gynecological cancers

- A huge percentage of women who are diagnosed with ovarian cancer have no prior history of the disease in their families
- Studies have shown that most of the women with ovarian cancer had early stage symptoms, yet in the U.S. 75% of women with ovarian cancer are diagnosed with late stage disease
- For the 25% who are detected early, the 5 year survival rate is greater than 90%
- Early detection is critical for long-term survival
- Ovarian cancer spreads quickly
- Common disorders, for example, digestive disorders, come and go and in time fade away altogether but ovarian cancer symptoms persist and gradually get worse.

So, ladies, here's what you need remember:

- No one knows your body better than you do and your body never lies
- Memorize the above list of symptoms
- Symptoms are the language your body uses to get your attention—listen to your body
- If you have symptoms that don't go away and worsen, after a few weeks, seek medical attention and insist on having:

  1 A CA125 blood test
  2 A pelvic examination

3 A vaginal ultrasound

o If you are diagnosed with ovarian cancer make sure you are treated by a gynecological oncologist

o Even if you are healthy and do not have ovarian cancer, never miss your annual gynecological check-up

o If you have a history of ovarian cancer or a strong history of breast cancer in your family, consider screening, genetic testing and treatment options—while you are still healthy.

You may find it interesting to hear that the question I was most asked on the journey, and since, is "How was 'it' discovered?"

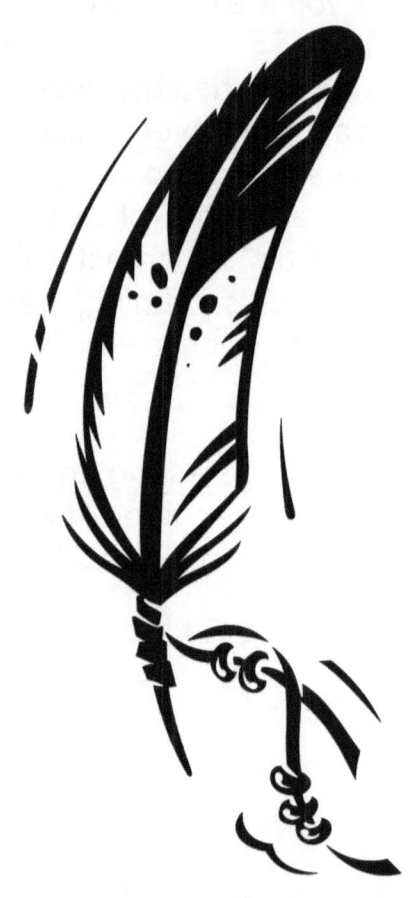

Spiritual evolution, communication with
spirit, celestial wisdom, truth & light.

PRAYERS, GOOD ENERGY & HEALING

I no longer differentiate between prayers, good energy and healing.

These days, there is no difference, for me, with what words, which language, or within which religious context (or no religion) prayers are said. It's all the same. For me there is one Great Spirit and 'Universal' energy. All roads lead to the same destination, the end result is the same.

Throughout the illness I was prayed for, by family, friends, loved ones, friends of friends and even total strangers, under the roofs of every kind of religious institution that exists, churches, mosques, synagogues, (in alphabetical order!) prayer groups, meditation groups, healing groups, people lit candles for me in their homes, they held me in their thoughts and in their hearts, they sent good wishes, good energy, distant healing, they did hands-on healing and surrounded me with love and light. No wonder I healed, I was truly blessed.

The common ground between all the prayer, good energy and healing that I was sent was the intention with which they were sent out to the Universe. As Gregg Braden explains, prayer is not about the words you say, when you pray, but about the feeling you have inside, when you are praying and about visualizing the prayer as already having been answered.

Each and every prayer, wish, request, particle of energy and thought was heard, came my way, was felt and took effect. There is no doubt in my mind that all the prayers, good energy and healing played a huge, significant and decisive role in my ultimate recovery. The power of all this prayer is engraved in my heart and my memory forever.

The infinite power and love of God or the Universe, (call it by any name you wish) was tangible. I felt that all things were possible. I knew I was not alone. It was clear that, when the time was right, I'd feel well again. I once read that God helps us not because of what we do, or don't do, but because of who He is. That feels right.

The feelings and emotions with which people prayed for me ignited the divine spark in me, and helped me to connect with and recognize the divine spark in people of all religious beliefs, persuasions and paths and it was clear that we are all one.

HELP ME!

I ask you to help me to accept what is happening
to me.
Help me to be strong when I feel fearful and
tired.
Help me to get out of bed and stay out for as
long as I can.
Help me to think positive thoughts.
Help me to see things differently:
Sick → challenged
Tired → need to rest
Afraid → all is well.

Dee

I PRAY . . .

LIVING IN THE MOMENT—NOW

Cancer teaches you that the life you once enjoyed is over and that there is no guarantee about your future. So, where does that leave you? Fortunately for you, it leaves you in the present—the very best and only place worth being. The moment, now, is the only time you can be sure of, because it's already in your hand.

I used to be a do, do, do person. Cancer taught me how to live in the moment and just 'be'. My relief was enormous. My life slowed down to the pace of a tortoise. All I could cope with was what I held in my hand. I no longer thought way into the future or made long range plans. I started living for today—fully—to the very kernel of my being, tomorrow really did mean 'another day' to me. Tomorrow ceased to exist for me until it became 'today'.

The cancer journey (even post cancer) can be a time of great fear. You fear the unknown, pain, suffering, not being able to cope, a recurrence of the illness and the list goes on. The one sure way to live without fear is to live in the now. Our minds can only hold one thought at a time. When you are totally present in everything you are doing, while you are doing it, you'll find that your whole focus is on what you are currently doing and, hey presto, you don't feel any fear.

I know this to be true. This doesn't mean that I don't feel fearful at times. I do. When I become aware of my fearfulness I do my utmost to bring myself back into present time consciousness and get back into the now—where I'm safe. Let me put it more simply . . . when I live 'mindfully' the rest doesn't seem to matter. I don't take it a day at a time, but rather, a moment at a time. For me, this is the secret of mental wellbeing. It's a stress-free, fear-free and serene place to be.

I can no longer muster extra excitement about specific days like holidays, anniversaries, or birthdays, because every single day is a special day for me now. Every day I wake up and feel good is a gift and I feel the same joy as others feel on 'special days'. **Today** is special.

Don't talk about doing things when you feel better than you do today or when you are older, or when this or that comes to pass—that time may never be yours to have. Talk, think and act now.

Even when I'm understandably anxious in the days preceding a scan or blood test, I still make it my mission to enjoy as much as possible, so as not to waste even one precious day or moment.

LETTING GO OF THE PAST
& THE FUTURE . . .

IT AIN'T OVER TILL IT'S OVER

So, you have just received your last chemotherapy treatment. You most likely feel a lot worse than you did after previous treatments quite simply because with each surgery, chemotherapy treatment and radiation session your immune system, your body and your strength take a massive beating, bashing and bruising. Now, you have finally made it to the last treatment, having more or less crawled to the finishing line of your journey and everyone is happy, relieved and excited that it's all over.

Well, hey, the only thing is that it's not over yet! It's over for everyone else but it's not over for you. It's so understandable that everyone feels that it's time to get back to 'normal' and that it's over at last. This has been a marathon for all your loved ones, carers, staunch supporters and 'sisters' too. What some people forget though is that after every other chemo session it took you between five to ten days to surface and gather together enough strength to participate, at the most minimal level, in everyday life. Does this last treatment not deserve at least that amount of time, acceptance and understanding too?

It can happen that there is an unspoken expectation that you should be well again now, able to cope and get on with life. But you can't! You're just not able. You feel so completely wiped out with exhaustion, your body aches, your system is filled with toxins, your immune system is smashed, your emotions still feel raw and you may even harbor personal disappointment that you aren't recovering quickly enough either. You can sense when someone calls and asks how you are that they now expect the reply "I feel a lot better" or "I feel great."

I was fortunate enough to have been warned about this stage of the journey by my chemo pal, Laura, who had already had cancer before we shared this cancer journey together. Long before treatments ended, she casually remarked one day, about it possibly taking at least six months after treatments finished, before I'd begin to feel like myself again. The information was stored in my brain that day, but the full understanding and the reality of it did not quite register.

Recovery is so slow that at times you wonder whether you are moving backwards instead of forwards. It's like taking two steps forward and one step back. It's a day at a time, an hour at a time, moment by moment. There definitely were times when I wondered whether I'd ever feel fully well, healthy and energetic again. The people who really loved me and cared were still there by my side, encouraging me, applauding me, praising my progress and just being there for me still—and how I needed them.

It took six months before I felt fairly well again, considering all I had been through. Now, it's been a year since the last chemo treatment and I feel I'm almost there. I didn't get my health back as it was pre cancer. I got something new. I'm grateful.

For me, staying well now means taking my wellness programme seriously, every single day. If for any reason I miss doing even one element of my programme for a day or two at most, I already start to feel unwell; the first symptom being serious tiredness, followed by an achy body and in quick succession low spirits. One just doesn't want to feel that unwell ever again!

HOW I FEEL NOW THAT TREATMENTS ARE OVER . . .

SEND IT BACK

It was time for a Shaman bonfire. I was three months post chemo and ready to clear cancer energy out of my body, my home and my life, forever.

I gathered together all the things that reminded me of the cancer journey and chucked them in the boot of my car.

I could feel the importance and significance of my mission, to me. I knew already as I drove to the site of the bonfire that I'd feel different once I'd offloaded these blatant reminders of cancer from my home and my life. It felt like another operation of sorts—cutting away and destroying the last visual reminders of cancer, that still clung and were daily reminders.

Setting up the bonfire was easy. It all felt so right. On to the fire I gleefully and joyfully threw my towels (reminders of my separation from the rest of the family in an effort to stay sterile and illness free), my bandanas (for obvious reasons!), the 'famous folder' (minus the documents, of course!) that I'd loyally carried (from doctor to doctor, from treatment to treatment, from check-up to check-up, from surgery to surgery, from scan to scan, from blood test to blood test and so on) for the last year, my pyjamas (reminders of time spent in bed) and anything else I'd found in my home that triggered cancer thoughts.

I sat on the ground, the sun beaming energy into my body, breathing in good health and gratitude, exhaling cancer, chemotherapy and illness. I was letting go. I watched all the reminders of cancer catch fire, burn and return to mother earth as ashes, never to arise again. As I watched I said, three times:

"I, Dee, return the cancer to Mother Earth, with infinite love and gratitude. I'm grateful for the gifts it brought and the lessons it taught me. Cancer is over and behind me now. I choose to move on without it. I openly, willingly and with great joy, embrace the next stage of my journey. My body is now healthy, well, able and strong. All is well in my world."

I waited till the fire had completely burned down and cancer was wiped from my space. As I got into my car, for the return journey home, with an empty boot, I felt my life was empty of cancer now too. I felt lighter. My relief felt physical as well as emotional. There was a large space in my life now that needed filling with new life, good health, joy and most of all gratitude.

I'M FINISHED WITH CANCER FOREVER . . .

THE GIFT OF CANCER

It is my opinion that all challenging situations in life come with gifts attached. There are two kinds of gifts that come with cancer. There is the type that comes in the post and the type that the Universe sends. Both are most welcome!

It could be difficult to see cancer as a gift from the Universe, at first. Only much later, when one has made lots of changes for the better and life feels so much more comfortable (as if it 'fits' you), can one recognize the gift. In time, you may even be grateful for it.

Do you think you'd have made all (or any) of the changes that you have made had you not done the cancer journey?

- o Would you be healthy in mind, body and spirit without the gift?
- o Would you still be plodding along in your old life, knowing that it was unhealthy on some, or all levels, but not making the effort to sort it out?
- o Would you still be burying pain and emotional issues in your body tissues and organs?
- o Would you have been emotionally strong enough to get out of unhealthy relationships?
- o Would you have learned to say "No?"
- o Would you have learned to let go and flow with life?

o Would you have been able to understand the impact and importance of the thoughts and words you send out to the Universe?

o Would you have been capable of taking responsibility for your own life, your health and your future?

o Would you ever have taken time to discover the joy of really, really having fun?

o Would you have learned to receive or would you have continued only giving?

o Would you have found balance in your life?

o Would you have found the inner peace and serenity that you now enjoy?

o Would you have learned to let go of the past and live in the now?

o Could you possibly have learned a fraction of what you learned (and lived) without the gift of the cancer journey from the Universe?

Let me hazard a guess? No!

The purpose of this gift is to get your attention—well, it certainly does that successfully—who wouldn't notice being whacked over the head with a 50kg hammer?! This gift shows you how to learn, heal and grow. How, and to what extent it shapes you, is entirely up to you.

You learn to let go, to forgive, to change, to appreciate everybody and everything in your life, you learn about gratitude, how to live in the moment, to take your health and wellness seriously, to 'be' and not just 'do' all the time, to be a better human being and have something more worthwhile to contribute to humanity. Most of all you learn to value the gift of your health, of each new day, of life and of feeling well, when you do.

With the gifts you now possess you'll have so much to offer any Champ who comes behind you on a similar journey. You'll be able to walk away from any situation or relationship, in your life, that is no longer healthy for you. You may feel at times that you are not as physically strong as you were pre-cancer but, you are much stronger (in a calm and gentle way) as a person, than before, and you most likely like it.

You have managed to stop wasting energy trying to please everyone, to quit saying 'yes' when you dream of saying 'no' and you know you'll never ever again waste a moment of your precious time doing anything you don't want to do.

You'll open each day like the precious and treasured gift that it is. You'll bathe in the joy of your newly awakened and strengthened mind, body and spirit. You may have had to face possible death, in order to value your life and live it fully, but now you do and that's all that matters. As Bernie Rhodes so wisely says "What really matters is not where you come from but where you are going."

CANCER BROUGHT ME MANY GIFTS . . .

BENEFITS

There is yet another kind of gift that comes with cancer, called 'benefits'. Are you aware that you may be entitled to some extra help at this time? When I was first informed, by the social worker at the chemo unit, that there were benefits available to me, I was deeply surprised. At that early stage I didn't think I needed any. Oh boy, did I learn in time the value of each one and how to be grateful for them.

Every country offers different help so let me share with you what was generously available to me:

o Free parking at the hospital for the entire year of treatments, surgeries, check-ups and tests

o Refunds on all transportation costs to and from the hospital, whether it was by taxi, bus or private car

o Our City Taxes were reduced to half for the duration of the illness

o The provision of a handicapped sticker for my car was a benefit I thought I'd never need, but it didn't take long for me to understand and value this gift

o Social Services generously paid me about $500 a month until the doctors declared me fit and well again o At the hospital I had access to every kind of free support I needed—social worker, psychologist, yoga, wig or hair-trimming and the list goes on.

I am very aware that these benefits didn't come about all by themselves. Champs who survived cancer before me saw the need for these benefits and on recovery made the effort to contribute and make the journey easier for the Champs coming along behind them. They made a difference (and how) by no doubt campaigning and working to ensure that people like me would have an easier journey. I had. Every time I pulled into a parking space near the door of the shopping centre, which helped save valuable and scarce energy that I needed for later, a wave of gratitude engulfed me. The benefits gave validation and recognition to the seriousness and challenge of the illness. I felt the compassion and consideration behind the benefits.

Most Champs who complete their journey have a burning desire to help and make a difference. No matter how small the effort you make, it will make a difference. If, in your country, there are no benefits like the few mentioned above, maybe you could work to make better benefits available for Champs like you. Not all women are good campaigners or may not feel well enough for it. Fear not, there are so many ideas to work on. You could donate an electric bed to the chemo unit, or more comfortable seats for the visitor's area, or treat the outstanding nursing team to a gift, or buy a nice picture for one of the bedrooms at the unit, or see what might be missing at the chemo unit—a television, a DVD, some books, games, a toaster—you'll know. If any of this is beyond you, you could offer support to another woman who is starting her journey, it can even be done effectively over the phone. Every time I pass the rooms I slept in, at the unit, after my surgeries, I send a silent prayer, blessing and healing to the Champs who currently occupy those beds.

The choices are endless and each and every one will be of benefit to someone—we only want to make a difference, after all, not change the world! Everyone has something to offer and that includes you.

BENEFITS AVAILABLE TO ME . . .

CANCER PROFILE

I've heard people talk about the 'cancer profile'. So, what does that mean? It's a profile, or certain personality type, that some people believe fits people who get cancer.

Some say that, in general, Champs are people who give all the time but are not as good at knowing how to receive; that they are people pleasers, who are at the bottom of their own list themselves most of the time; people who bury their emotional pain in their body tissues; who are angry with life or others or themselves but hide it; or people who hide various types of pain, due to past traumas, in specific body organs. I'm not saying that this is true. I'm just sharing the possibility with you.

Champs often keep going with a certain relationship, lifestyle, behavior or direction, even when it feels completely and totally wrong for them, until one day their body screams "No more." Then, there is no longer a choice, cancer stops them and they finally have to address issues, make changes, let go, learn and start taking care of themselves.

Champs learn, the hard way, about:

o Receiving, and not just giving
o Setting boundaries, saying "no" to others and "yes" to themselves
o Forgiveness being a gift they bestow on themselves

- o Balance
- o Putting themselves first
- o Letting go of everything that doesn't resonate with them
- o Getting out of toxic situations of every kind— including relationships
- o Letting go of blame and taking responsibility
- o 'Being' as well as 'doing'
- o Operating from the heart and not just the head
- o Thinking the kind of thoughts that will form the reality they dream of
- o Living more joyfully and planting themselves firmly in their own power.

All these changes do not make the Champ selfish and inconsiderate, but rather fill her up in the most positive and constructive way, so that she now has so much more to offer and give, as opposed to running on empty most of the time. She is now ready to live life on her own terms. She is now capable of being a healthy, fully functional member of society, making a difference and doing whatever it is she was born to do, or always dreamed of doing.

The average Champ may once have fitted the cancer profile but that was her 'old song'. She's now singing her heart out to her very own composition—the ballad that tells the exciting and vibrant story of her new life, as created and directed by herself.

MY PROFILE, AS I SEE MYSELF NOW . . .

THINGS TO GET USED TO

At the start of the journey a Champ has many difficult elements to get used to. That's why if you are supporting, helping or sharing the journey with a Champ, the early days of the journey (the first two months in particular) are the time when your support is most needed and valued. The Champ, at this stage, is most likely floundering, lost and overwhelmed by the number of changes in her life and the speed at which they occur.

Changes . . . ? Yes.

There is cancer in your body. You are no longer healthy. You face some, or all, of chemotherapy, radiotherapy and surgery. Unpleasant and painful side-effects lie in wait. You are about to lose all your hair. Hospitals, doctors, tests, scans, ultrasounds, check-ups and blood-tests are now part of your everyday reality.

You are no longer in charge or control of your own life. Your life no longer revolves around your schedule but rather around cancer. Wellness takes a front seat, work and everything else is now in the back seat. Life as you have known it to date no longer exists.

Waiting becomes a regular feature—waiting for tests, waiting for test results, waiting for doctor's appointments, waiting to recover from side-effects, waiting, waiting and more waiting.

There is a myriad of emotional upheaval. You face fears. There are endless tears.

You will need to start asking for help and as a result, you'll learn to receive.

What a Champ most needs at this earthquake eruptive time is support, hugs, listening, sympathy, practical help and friendship.

Keep in touch with a Champ, no matter what. Always start with:

o How are you?
o How do you feel?
o What can I do to help you?

Having completed the journey, I can say that the following elements were the most challenging for me:

o The sheer intensity of the exhaustion and trying to function, heal and stay alive on zero energy
o The length of time it took me to recover and the endlessness of it all
o Letting go of my old life and all that it meant to me was crushing
o Not being able to be the Mum I'd usually been to my children was devastating
o Not being able to live a 'normal' life for so long was hard
o The feeling of being separate from the rest of the world was lonely

o Not being able to 'keep up' was new and unwelcome

o The side-effects of chemotherapy, the excruciating pain, the loss of my hair and so many body organs was devastating

o Being house-bound for so many days at a time was restrictive

o Waking up in the morning with plans and moments later having to accept that I didn't have the energy to execute them was frustrating

o The transition from looking good to feeling good took time

o Barely recognizing myself when I looked in the mirror was a shock

o Letting go of people who I thought would be there for me, but weren't, was the stuff grief is made of.

I thought I knew how to wait until I got into this 'game'—now I really and truly know how to wait. I understand, accept and have learned that particular lesson very nicely, thank you!

GETTING USED TO _____
WAS HARD FOR ME . . .

FIRST HAIR CUT

The morning of my first post-chemo hair cut had arrived. I felt 100% sure that it was the right day to proceed. It's a big decision to have your hair cut when you have been bald for so long. You wonder whether you should wait a little longer, let your hair grow a bit more, let it get a bit thicker and stronger first. Finally, you decide to go ahead and it's a big event for you.

I felt happy and joyful. I relished every moment of my time at the salon, not having been for a shampoo and hair-cut for over a year. It almost felt like unfamiliar territory.

Sitting at the sink having my hair washed sent huge waves of emotion rushing through me. Tears welled in my eyes. I knew I'd come full circle. Had I ever before even considered how fortunate I'd been to pop off to the hairdresser every six weeks and have anything of my choosing done to my hair? No, I hadn't. This was something else to add to my ever-lengthening gratitude list.

The hairdresser was kind and listened as I explained that I was post-chemo and this was my first cut. I was totally unprepared for the level of kindness and compassion that followed. The other two young hairdressers abandoned their posts and all three hairdressers encircled my chair.

As the hairdresser cut my hair, his colleagues watched intently, they asked questions about the cancer journey in an open, relaxed and non-fearful way. They listened and hung on my every word. They were interested in my story and, considering their young age, I was impressed and moved.

The hairdresser followed my wishes to a tee. He and his colleagues wished me well as I left and I knew they really meant it. It had been a warm and relaxing experience. I was grateful for their compassion, consideration and caring.

I thought about the women who complain that their hair is too short, too curly, too straight, too oily, too wavy . . . get over yourselves girls, just be glad you have hair at all! Instead of complaining, just enjoy what you've got, give thanks for it and save your energy for having fun and living life to the full instead.

P.S. It may be worth noting that hair may not have any pigment after chemotherapy so the first time you try to colour your hair, post chemo, it may not 'take' properly or fully. In other words, your hair may not turn out the same as the colour on the box of hair colour! It usually takes three or four sessions of colouring before your hair colours accurately and evenly.

Also, it's good to remember that your hair grows back in the same way as a baby's. This means that it may grow in all directions and unevenly. Just think of the average two-year-old's 'all over the shop' hair! You may need to use gel to 'control' it for the first few months. Your hair may not grow at the same speed as it grew at before you were ill. Growing your hair may take longer than you think.

THE JOY OF HAVING HAIR AGAIN . . .

RECOVERY

"We have the power to create in our world what we imagine in our belief," Gregg Braden.

You are the one who has been extremely ill so it makes sense then that you are the one who has to work hard to recover your wellness and perfect health again. It will mark a significant turning point for you, on the cancer journey, when you admit to yourself that you are responsible for your own recovery and that survivors really do take charge.

Recovery is a very slow process. If you have had surgery, chemotherapy and radiation your body has, in fact, been cut, poisoned and burned! You have been to hell and back, so it may take a long time for your body to recover from this severe trauma. Be gentle and patient with yourself. When you are in recovery you have to let go of deadlines and learn to flow with it. You cannot set time limits to this. There is no special place or stage you should be at by a particular date. You'll be well and truly recovered only when you are and not a moment before. You may recover slower or quicker than someone else who had the same surgeries and treatments as you did—it's very individual. Give yourself all the time you need to heal—even if, at times, it feels like it's taking forever.

When months have rolled by and you feel like there are still so many things you can't yet do, the trick is to remind yourself about all the things you actually **are** able to do and stop focusing on the activities that you are, meanwhile, unable to master. All will be well, in time, when the time is right.

My absolute belief in the concept of my body being a perfect healing organism, helped me to stay strong, even when it felt that my reality wasn't quite matching up. Months after treatments ended I was still exhausted, looked unhealthy, had to plan extra activity around lots of rest, still needed help from all my loyal carers and supporters, still had very short hair, nails that weren't growing, an almost non-existent immune system, a very dull brain, hearing that was far from sharp, blurred vision, pain in my feet day and night, blood test results that showed every organ in my body was strained and the list goes on.

There is no doubt in my mind that affirmations were one of my most useful tools during recovery time. It sounds easy and it really is simple. All day, every day, I would say the recovery-affirming sentences below, over and over again:

- o My body is a perfect healing organism
- o I am healthy, happy and healed
- o The nerve endings in my hands and feet are in perfect working order
- o I am a cancer survivor.

This was a very lonely time for me. The framework of treatments (and everything that went with that) was gone, I was supposed to be healing but I still felt so weak, tired, drained and anything but healthy. Sometimes I felt very sad and depressed. It seemed like the whole process was never-ending. At one point I fell into a deep black hole of dark depression, for about three weeks. I had no idea how I was ever going to save myself.

It can be a bit scary when you realize that you are now finished treatments, you won't be going to the hospital as often, the oncologist has done everything he can to cure you and you are on your own in terms of healing. Fear not, there is so much you can do to help yourself—things you can do that will really make an enormous difference to how you feel on a daily basis and to how you recover and heal. I have repeated this same list in the chapter about Long-term Survivors (page 193) and the Wellness chapter (page 99). That will give you some idea of how important, significant and truly effective I feel self-help is. In this way you can be an active participant in your own healing. It takes a mammoth **daily** effort, and lots of patience, but I assure you that, in time, it pays off to:

- o Eat a healthy diet of fresh, organic, non-processed food
- o Drink at least eight glasses of filtered water daily

o   Exercise, at least walking
o   Get enough rest at night and I'd personally recommend a nap as well
o   Be in your own power
o   Meditate and practice Yoga or Reiki
o   Drink fresh, organic vegetable juices
o   Say affirmations, like those listed above, or make up your own
    (See also the Affirmations chapter, page 56)
o   Make time for breathing exercises
o   Take vitamins and supplements recommended by a certified Chinese Medicine Practitioner or Naturopath.

All of the above will strengthen you in such a way that healing can take place.

Why not take your recovery to a different level altogether—quite simply, assume that you are recovering and that you are already well! Direct your emotions to believe that it's already a fact. Believe it to be so.

If you feel disheartened about the slow pace of your recovery and fear that you may never be well again, you could talk to a friend who supported you on the journey, your chemo pal, your social worker or your oncologist. Feel all your feelings. If you feel disappointed, sad or upset in any way, have a good cry, it's a wonderful release.

Try not to see yourself as a victim at this important stage of your journey. You are not a victim, you are a beautiful soul, whose body has been severely traumatized and wounded—you have survived the ordeal till now, don't give up, you are almost there and the worst is already behind you. You are doing much better than you may realize.

Accept the uncertainty of recovery, there will be good hours followed by weak and exhausting ones; further on there will be two good days followed by a day when you have to spend hours in bed; later still, you'll get through a good week when you feel relatively 'normal' and then you'll hit what may feel like an all time low, you'll question your progress, your health, your future and your very existence. Give yourself time. Everyone is different and you are unique, so take as long as **you** need. It took me a year before I felt fully well and truly healed. Even at that, I didn't get back the endless energy I had pre-cancer. I got a new life, new health, a new chance, it's different and I'm grateful.

You'll find that you have not yet finished learning lessons just yet. In this recovery phase learning can happen at an even faster pace than when you were in treatments.

It's so exciting when you no longer need to use anti-bacterial soap, or when you don't have to rinse your mouth with salt+bicarbonate of soda several times a day (to avoid mouth ulcers). It feels so good when you can go out for an evening and feel energetic enough to enjoy yourself and stay awake till the end of the evening! You may just cry the first time you look in the mirror and realize you no longer look sick or have 'the chemo look'. Imagine the freedom and elation you'll feel the first time you have enough hair, all over your head, to go out and about without your wig! Little by little you'll begin to believe that 'it' may be over at last and you'll begin to see a welcome bright light at the end of the long, dark and winding tunnel.

During your recovery you will still need lots of love, support and help. There is no need to keep apologizing to others about not feeling well just yet, or not being able to keep up. Everyone else knows and accepts that, it's abundantly clear to all—you are possibly the only one who needs convincing!

o Take full responsibility for your recovery
o Believe in your recovery
o Understand that recovery is a slow process and that it takes time
o Do everything you can to help yourself— whatever it takes
o Listen to your body, it knows best what you need at this time
o Accept any offer of help, you may still need it!

MY RECOVERY . . .

6 MONTHS DOWN THE ROAD

"You will be lost before you are found," Helen Exley.

In the same way that we see a change and a leap forward in the development of a baby at six weeks, three months and six months, so it was with my recovery.

At six months my body felt a bit fitter and stronger. My muscle tone and skin were beginning to feel a bit more recognizable to me. My eyebrows and eyelashes had returned and how happy I was to see these mostly undervalued body parts back in place. My nails still barely grew and only needed trimming once every three to four weeks. I had put on a little weight.

I had more of a spring in my step, as opposed to plodding and dragging. I was capable of more exercise. I could stay up all day but knew that a daily nap would keep my energy level stable over a longer period of time. Tiredness, sometimes complete and total exhaustion, can go on for months after treatments have ended . . . and did at times.

I no longer thought about my CA125 level all the time. I believed it would balance itself, in time. Healthy, well, able and strong fit me a bit more comfortably. My brain function and short-term memory were improving. I felt a lot less fuzzy, spaced and lost.

The buzzing/numb/pain sensation in my feet (damage to the nerve endings in my feet due to chemo drugs—Raynaud Syndrome—google it!) no longer triggered fearful cancer thoughts in my mind every time I put a foot on the ground. Life was beginning to feel more 'normal' again.

Normal also means busy. It will take a huge effort to keep your life at a size and style that 'fits' you—to live mindfully as opposed to mindless rushing around. It can be hard to find time for wellness, and to live in the way you feel you need to in order to stay healthy, because life is life, you are either part of it or you are not. There are parts of life that you can't evade, escape or ignore.

I try to do the important things that need to be done, early in the morning, while I still have energy. Even if I nap in the middle of the day, I may not have a lot of energy after it, for the remainder of the day.

Feeling depressed, low or lost can follow the initial joy and exuberance of being finished chemo. You knew your pre-chemo life. Chemo itself had a very definite framework and cycle—you were busily in it and didn't need to think or act on your life as such. Now you are alone. You don't want to go back and you are not quite sure how to go forward to a new life either. You know you don't want the life you had pre-cancer, yet you may not be sure enough, well enough or energetic enough to go after a different life at the moment. There are days when you feel like a prisoner doing time for a crime you didn't commit! You feel you don't fit in. You want to go away somewhere and be alone. You want to escape. You try desperately to hold on tightly and not allow yourself to fall any deeper into the bottomless abyss of darkness that lies below, knowing that you would have to work so hard to climb back out of there. On such days I look at the photo that was taken of me on what I remember was the worst day of the entire chemo journey. I can hardly believe the unrecognizable woman in the photo is me. I feel pity, compassion and love for this person in the photo. She moves me to tears. I marvel at how far she has come and I know she is going to make it. I bring everything back to gratitude and things change immediately. I pull my focus back to the basics of wellness—water, food, rest, exercise and being in my own power (and the correct quantity, quality and frequency of each). I make sure I get to do every element of my wellness programme every day until, in a matter of days, I'm more on track again.

You may not feel quite as connected to some people as you once did. That is understandable. The cancer journey has changed you. They may not quite understand who you are now, because of where you have been, and you can't expect them to.

You may have a strong urge to take a really good holiday—to spend, eat out, relax, enjoy and catch up on all the fun you have missed out on in the last year or more. Taking a good holiday, preferably with someone whose company is restful and fun, is an excellent idea, once you get the 'all clear' from your oncologist. There is nothing more therapeutic than a great holiday and lots of fun.

You may have an overwhelming urge to spring-clean your house, de-junk, give things away that no longer suit the new you, and generally give your home a 'shake-up'. It's a wonderful idea to do this as it shifts all the old, sick, stuck energy out of your home and you can feel the lightness, freshness and movement of the new.

The post-chemo months are a time of great change. You are no longer sick and huge awareness floods in now that your entire focus and energy are no longer laser-pointed solely on your physical wellbeing. Don't feel the need to apologize to anyone about changes you have made or are making. You can explain why you are making the changes you are making, but without the apology side of it. This is who you are now and who you must remain in order to stay healthy and alive. Yes. You get to redefine love, life, goals, time, friendship, making a difference, what you want from your life (not someone else's), fear and flowing with life. You are now concerned about 'fixing' yourself and others can do the same for themselves.

You will become more comfortable and articulate about saying things you want to say, without the intention of hurting anyone.

Forgiveness will creep into your life. You will allow it to happen because you are ready. You see things differently and are open to the idea that anyone can make a mistake (including you!) and deserves a second chance.

I'm beginning to feel more capable, sure and free. I feel I can make a difference. Doing what I was born to do seems more attainable.

As you get healthier and stronger the phone calls to your chemo pal may become less frequent. The connection between you is still strong. You'll call on instinct these days. You'll just know when your pal could do with a call, from you, so you'll listen and be there for her. She will do the same for you.

Your oncologist's role is to cure the cancer, wellness is up to you and it's a full time job. Hopefully, by now, you have really gripped how important your daily wellness programme is. Healers and alternative people will guide you about diet, exercise, supplements, emotional changes and energy shifts. When people ask and I tell them about my current eating programme (and the various foods I no longer eat like dairy, red meat, white flour products and sweet things), they invariably ask "What else is there to eat?" I can assure you that there is such an abundance of fresh, tasty, unprocessed and nourishing food available, no matter where you live or what your budget—yes. It's all just a matter of priority. Remember it's all about you and your wellness. Take time to do what you know you need to do in order to stay well. Letting go of anything that's not important leaves you free time, energy and effort to focus on the importance of wellness and restoring your health.

I feel infinite love and gratitude for all the dear loved ones and friends who are still by my side, listening and supporting, constantly concerned and caring. I'll be eternally grateful and will never forget one act of support or effort to hold me up.

Let's not forget that by the time you are six months down the road, post chemo, that you will most likely be about to face your third round of blood tests and visit to your oncologist. Needless to add, the dreaded CA125 (ovarian cancer marker) blood test results also need to be faced. You have no doubt realized that it doesn't get easier as time goes on! The fear factor remains the same. You'll pass nights when you appear to be asleep but your mind is wide awake, filled with fear and dread. All logic tells you it's an unreasonable fear, but the terror still grips you and even if you don't want to, you still feel it. Once fear takes root, the boundaries of your mind give way to your wildest fears. You drag out of bed in the morning, totally exhausted, worn out, tired and still fearful, ready to start all over again—after all, today is a new day, a new start and new choices.

It's good to look back, learn and let go. I've changed. I'm comfortable with who I am now. I feel stronger about making wiser choices. I feel quietly confident now as I stand firmly in my own space, surrounded by my guides, angels, loved ones, lots of love, light and peace.

6 MONTHS LATER . . .

THE ONE YEAR MILESTONE

You've finally made it to the one year milestone. I'm talking, of course, about a year since your surgeries and treatments finished. It could well be about twenty months since your 'story' started. It's an amazing achievement! You may feel like you have climbed Mount Everest. Those who do, are fit and healthy, when they climb the highest mountain. You have been weak, energy-less, exhausted, in pain and a far cry from perfect health when you successfully climbed your highest mountain. You can feel so eternally proud and infinitely grateful for having come this far. Make sure you celebrate accordingly!

So, how do you feel? By now you probably feel healthy, strong, energetic and pain-free. It feels so good to be able to wake up free of pain and tiredness, to be able to do the ordinary things, to be able to drive when you want to, to be able to go out any time you choose because you feel well enough to do so. It's pure, undiluted joy.

You will note, that I haven't mentioned about your life being 'back' to normal again. That's because there is no going back, only forward! You most likely wouldn't want to go back anyway to the life that gave you cancer. You have changed so much on every level, learned so many lessons, let go of so much emotional baggage, disentangled yourself from many toxic situations (and possibly people), that your old life would most likely no longer 'fit' you anyway.

It's obvious to you at this stage that wellness, and doing what you need to do in order to stay well, is a full time job. Wellness is now a firm fixture at the top of my daily list. Taking care of my wellness comes first. I finally got it and made the necessary changes.

Taking care of 'me' now involves:

o Doing Reiki, Lifeline technique, being mindful, breathing exercises or all when I wake up in the morning
o Saying affirmations, such as,

1. My body is healthy, well, able and strong
2. I'm a cancer survivor
3. My body is a perfect healing organism
4. I am healthy, happy and healed

o Drinking about eight to ten glasses of water daily
o Going to the gym twice a week and walking on the other days
o Drinking organic vegetable juices
o Reading some inspirational material
o Eating fresh organic food
o Connecting with loved ones, either by text, call, mail or visit
o Having fun!
o Journaling

o Meditating
o Making a difference in at least one life daily
o Giving thanks and gratitude for just about everything—having a strong gratitude attitude
o Laughing, sitting down, napping, hugging, doing nothing!
o There is no doubt in my mind that the basics of healthy living are water, food, exercise, rest and being in your own power—each in the correct quantity, quality and frequency. If I begin to feel unwell, I go back to these basics and once I get enough of each I begin to feel well again (See Darren Weissman's book, The Power of Infinite Love and Gratitude—The Lifeline Technique).

The concept of every day, every hour, every minute and every second counting is not just something I know, it's something I do! I set goals, make plans and dream.

o Love has replaced all other emotions including sadness and disappointment.
o I have been given a second chance at life. I ask myself, "Why?"
o What am I supposed to be doing now? Doing more of? Doing less of? Not doing at all?
o How can I make a difference?
o Am I living my life on terms that are comfortable for me?

o Are there further changes to make?
o Is my soul singing?
o Do I use my time wisely?

Letting go of everything that's no longer important to me frees up lots of energy for living, enjoying and staying healthy.

I've learned to live life to the full between the oncology check-ups. Apart from the few days prior to a check-up when, without a shadow of a doubt, I feel anxious, nervous, worried and fearful, I forget about it all, as best I can, and get on with the more important business of living and enjoying life, every day.

You may think you have changed but have you really?

o How good are you at saying "no?"
o How busy is your life?
o Have you allowed yourself to be sucked back into the 'madness' already?
o How tired do you feel?
o Do you get enough rest?
o Are you at the top of your own list?
o How much time do you devote to your wellness every day?
o Do you think, feel and behave differently?
o Have you got rid of everything that, for you, was toxic, in your life?

It's clearer than ever to me that everything that happens in life happens in Divine Order, in other words, that everything happens at the right time, in the right way and in the right order.

It may throw you completely off balance if you suddenly find you feel low, depressed or sad. That is perfectly normal, from time to time. I wager a guess that if you stop to think for a minute and examine your life-style, you'll conclude that you have been doing too much and are quite simply exhausted. Take a few days to retreat, rest, relax and regroup. You'll find that in a matter of days you'll feel much better, if not wonderful again. If, on the other hand, you can't seem to shake off these feelings, after a few weeks, seek professional help.

A year after treatments have finished you realize that you are capable of looking upon the devastating, debilitating and challenging process you have just survived as something you can be grateful for in certain ways. One wouldn't choose it of course, but having completed the journey (even involuntarily!), you'll be the first to admit that you have learned, healed and grown on all levels—mind, body and spirit. You are prepared in ways, that no other experience in your life could have prepared you, for the next stage of your life and any future 'curve balls' that might shoot across your path!

P.S. Have fun . . . lots of!

12 MONTHS LATER . . .

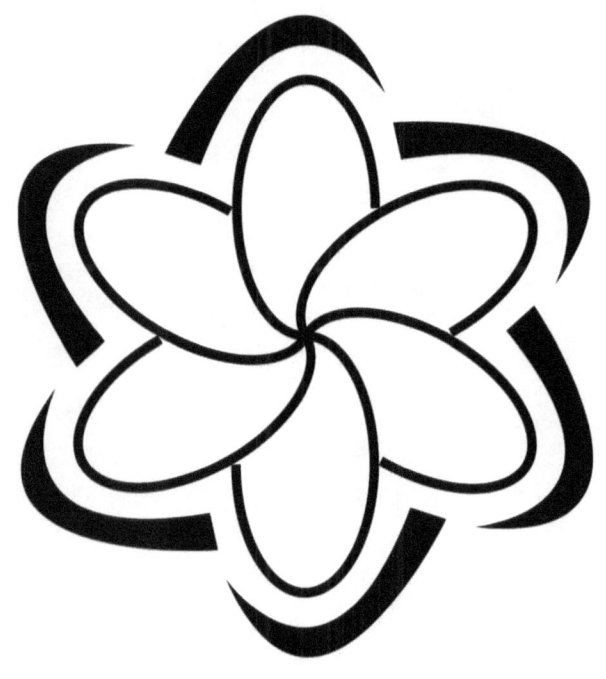

Celebration, beauty, summer, life!

GYM JUDGEMENT

I arrived for my first session at the gym with the pre-conceived notion that I'd be greeted by a lycra-clad personal trainer closely resembling the incredible hulk. Not only was my first illusion of the day shattered on meeting him but it was also my first lesson in non-judgment, for that day.

I was greeted warmly and without as much as a hint of super-fit arrogance. In front of me stood an 'old soul', aged twenty-eight! We chatted easily as I started my training. Yet again I knew I was not alone, that the Universe was with me all the way on this gym experience too. My trainer understood all about cancer. His Mum had died, from cancer, two years previously. She'd been given three months to live and had survived for seven years. There was no part of cancer that he hadn't experienced and that he didn't understand or respect. This was turning into an experience that felt so harmonious and right for me.

I'd never been to the gym before and had somehow thought (wrongly) that the gym was for already ultra-fit people. Illusion number two shattered and non-judgment lesson two learned. If I could learn to lift weights as fast as I was learning about non-judgment, then things were looking good!

I stole a quick look around and noticed that most of the people there were around my own age.

Without even asking, it became clear that lots of the people were there because, like me, they had waited till life whacked them with a 50kg mallet over the head before they really sat up, listened and started making changes.

To my utter amazement I survived a full hour at the gym that day. My third illusion of the day was shattered and my last lesson in non-judgment sank in. Before starting at the gym I was certain that I'd only be able for about ten minutes on my first day—mistake. I had visions of myself being carried out of there on a stretcher—mistake! The biggest mistake was forgetting that we are truly capable of so much more than we give ourselves credit for and we are much stronger than we realize.

I enjoyed every second of my first hour at the gym. I knew I'd be sticking with this. I'd slunk in there so unsure of myself and came out brim full of energy.

P.S. Six months later I feel the need to encourage everyone to exercise. There were days when I dragged myself to the gym, feeling I should possibly have cancelled—with my energy level hitting the floor and my mood dragging not too far behind. One hour later I'd skip out of the gym, oozing energy, bouncing and brimming with zest for life, for the rest of the day and at least the two following days.

For me it's not about looking good but about feeling good. My body is now strong. Much more important than all of that is the awareness that my mind is strong. The gym taught me that I'm capable of so much. I'm capable of doing more, enduring more, being more and I am definitely able.

MY NEW EXERCISE PLAN . . .

LESSONS LEARNED

Earth school is a pretty tough school to learn your lessons in, but cancer takes learning to a whole new level. Cancer is a wake-up call. It's about learning difficult lessons the hard way, quickly. By quickly I mean, over the relatively short time-span of the illness, as opposed to over the period of an entire lifetime.

Pre-cancer you may have felt, without giving it a lot of focused thought, that you were in a 'great place' emotionally, spiritually and physically. You may have thought that learning in this lifetime was going well for you.

Cancer stops you in your tracks and even if, at first, you question "Why me?" in time you'll turn your question around to "What am I supposed to be learning here?"

Whether you set out to learn through the cancer journey or not, it will happen anyway. You will learn, heal and grow to an extent that you could never have imagined was possible. It will help you to view cancer as a gift and possibly, in time, even with gratitude.

I learned to say no to others and yes to me.

I learned not to be part of anything that doesn't resonate with me—whether it's food, lifestyle, work, behavior or even people.

I learned to put wellness first because no plan in life can come to fruition in my life if I'm not healthy.

I learned to live in the 'now'.

I learned to let go and flow with things.

I learned to trust the Universe as if my life depends on it and it does!

I learned to sit down, or lie down, long before I might fall down, from exhaustion.

I learned to listen to my mind, my body and my soul and actually hear their message.

I learned that everything in life and the Universe is in a state of constant change.

I learned that I'm far stronger and more capable than I had initially realized.

I learned that all challenging situations in life come with gifts attached.

I learned that before God sends you on a mission He first provides you with the appropriate tools you'll need to successfully complete your challenge.

I learned to give gratitude for everything.

I learned that we are not the ones in charge, or control, of our lives.

I learned that curing and healing are not the same.

I learned that my thoughts and my words create my reality.

I learned that death is not to be feared, but 'not living' is.

I learned that if you are in any relationship (either personal, work related, family, or whatever) that's not working, you need to either fix it or get out.

I learned that every day is a special day—and that includes today!

I learned to choose carefully, how and with whom I spend my precious and very valuable time, from now on.

I learned that my life is in my own hands—I need to take responsibility for it, always.

I learned that every end is also a new beginning.

I learned that when our e-motions are not in motion, we get sick.

I learned that forgiving others is a gift I bestow on myself.

I learned that wellness doesn't have a price, it's priceless.

I learned how to slow down.

I learned the joy of yet another therapy—retail!

I learned that conventional medicine is necessary, alternative medicine is essential, they go hand in hand.

I learned the importance and value of fun, joy, celebration, laughter and enjoyment.

I learned that, no matter how bad yesterday was, today is a new day.

I learned that every day is a choice and I need to make that choice every day.

I learned that there is a time for 'doing' but I must also make time for 'being'.

I learned that doing or having anything that is not good for me is not a treat.

I learned that meditation helps me to hear the answers that lie between two heart-beats.

I learned to receive as well as give.

I learned to ask for help when I need it.

I learned to see, not imperfect people, but rather, perfect souls.

I learned to accept, with gratitude, the love that is being offered to me, in the way and on the terms in which it is being offered.

I learned that we are all connected, we are all one and we are all part of the Divine Matrix.

I learned that a thought is just a thought and can be changed.

I learned that it's okay to feel low, or angry, or sad, or tearful from time to time.

I learned that it's worth it to take time to breathe properly

I learned that food and nutrition are miracle medicine.

I learned that mind, body and soul are interconnected. I can't heal one in isolation from the others. All three need to be worked on for complete healing.

I learned that statistics are just that, statistics—I don't have to be one of them.

I learned that no matter how hard I think my situation is, there are many millions of people whose lives are more difficult than mine—without question, I can find many reasons to be grateful.

I learned that stress causes illness and I'm too blessed to be stressed.

I learned to get into the driver's seat of my life, where I plan to stay.

I learned that when I feel tired, it's best not to fight it, just sleep.

I learned, with the help of Darren Weissman's book 'The Power of Infinite Love and Gratitude', not to own the illness, i.e. not to say "My cancer" or "I have cancer."

I learned that daily exercise helps to keep me healthy, well, able and strong.

I learned to let go of the past and move on without it.

I learned that there is always a choice and I get to do the choosing.

I learned that 'feeling good' leaves 'looking good' in the shade!

I learned to feel my feelings—all of them.

I learned to express my emotions and not store them away.

I learned that no matter what I see on the news, the world is filled with loving, kind, compassionate, generous, helpful, special and wonderful human beings. When I set my mind on this, these are the people I meet.

I learned that I am not alone.

I learned that doctors can cure me but healing is up to me.

I learned to listen, interpret and understand the sensations in my body and respond accordingly.

257

I learned that recovery is a process (a long one!) and it takes time (lots of!).

I learned to listen & hear, to see & know, to believe & act and to trust & let go.

I learned that life is best lived one day at a time.

I learned that when I can't keep up that I don't have to—so I don't.

I learned that being proactive about monitoring, check-ups, doctor's visits, tests and scans saves lives.

I learned that work on wellness is not a life-sentence but, rather, a way of life.

I learned that everything in the Universe is in Divine order, which means, that everything happens in the right way, in the right order and at the right time.

I learned that the body is a perfect healing organism.

I learned that when you set your mind on healing that the Universe lays everything you need to make it come to pass, at your feet. All you need to do is to 'send it out there, let go, trust and wait'.

I learned from The Lifeline Technique, that the 5 basics of health are: food, water, exercise, rest and being in your own power—and the correct quantity, quality and frequency of each.

I learned that prayer is not about the words you say but about the feeling in your heart when you say those words.

I learned that I no longer need to be all things to all people. I'm content just being me.

I learned that I don't need (nor is it right for me) to do anyone else's journey for them. Their journey is theirs and mine is mine. My role is to love and support them with great compassion, but not to do their journey for them.

I learned that 'now' is the only time there is.

I learned that other people don't need to change, I need to change.

I learned to never, never, ever, ever give up, there is always hope.

And wait . . . in a nutshell . . . here's what I know for sure now . . . it all boils down to

- ✓ Not doing anything that doesn't resonate with you or feel right for you.
- ✓ Living joyfully . . . laughing, having fun, and doing what you feel passionate about that makes your soul sing.

LOVE THE LESSON!

Knowing that I make my own reality,
Help my light to shine brighter than ever at this
time,
So that my learning may be a catalyst for change
in the lives of others,
Help me to remember that I chose this
challenge long before I was born,
That it is part of my journey, my soul's
evolvement.
It's just another lesson.
I embrace it with gratitude.

Dee

I LEARNED THAT . . .

AND ANOTHER THING

It's now, sixteen months since my journey ended, that I can answer the question "How are you?" with the reply "I feel wonderful" and really mean it. I finally feel healthy, happy and healed.

It was a conscious choice to let go of cancer. I felt that I was holding on to 'it' as opposed to 'it' holding me. I decided I didn't want to carry a ball and chain around with me 24/7 anymore. Cancer, is no longer my whole life, it's just part of it. I refuse to drown in it or drag anyone else into the swamp with me.

I now understand that my body is my best friend. It loves me unconditionally. No matter what, it endures and does its very best for me, each and every day. I'll treat this treasured friend with the respect and kindness it truly deserves from now on.

There is no magic formula for surviving the cancer journey. You will get it as right as possible by listening to your body, tuning into your gut feeling and doing what you know in your heart is right for you, for now. So, whether you chose to go the conventional, or the alternative path, or combine both (as I did), you have to feel 100% comfortable with your decisions and treatments—if you don't, you can be sure that your body and your spirit are trying desperately to tell you something, so listen up.

From here on out I know my life is about trust. I need to trust the Universe, my medical team, the love and support that surround me and most of all, me! I know that no matter what happens that I'm held in the palm of God's hand and there is no safer place to be.

It's very clear to me now who really supports me, who truly loves me and who deserves a seat in the circle of support that surrounds me and keeps me buoyant. I no longer allow people who are not genuinely there for me to take up a valuable place in the circle, that someone who loves me unconditionally, deserves to occupy. I have learned to let go, with love and gratitude, and move on.

I'm happier, in love with life, enjoy more, feel more peaceful and live, very consciously, in the moment these days—with the odd dark day thrown in for balance! On the dark days I remind myself that O/C stands for 'Ovarian Cancer' but also for 'overcome'!

OVERCOME!

May you be swathed in love
May you be protected and healed
Trust that all is as it's meant to be
Be assured that you are exactly in the right place
at the right time
Breathe in health, serenity, tranquility and peace
Exhale anything that for you, today, is toxic
Feel and bathe in the love that surrounds you
Give gratitude for all your endless gifts
Relax, laugh, enjoy and have fun!

Dee

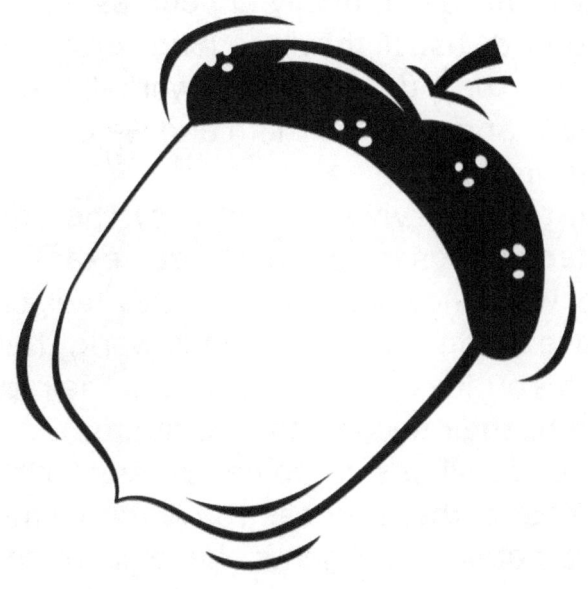

"The creation of 1,000 forests is in one acorn."
Ralph Waldo Emerson

LONG-TERM SURVIVIAL

"What doesn't kill us makes us stronger," Friedrich Nietzsche.

I feel that survivor's stories and experiences can never be valued highly enough as a guide and inspiration to us. If they are long-term survivors then what they do obviously works! We should look, learn and emulate them and we can be long-term survivors too.

Long-term survivors often defy the odds and have many things in common. Let's examine what they do, what they don't do, how they feel, changes they have made, how their minds work, their daily wellness routines, their fears and their general attitude to their second chance at life.

How do survivors get to be survivors in the first place? Most of them choose conventional medicine and alternative treatments, hand in hand. They are proactive in their own healing. They have a support network—of people who also believe they will make it. They have a strong will to survive. They have learned to let go of anger and other negative emotional issues.

Long-term survivors understand that no matter how hard they try, that they are not the ones in charge or control of their lives. They know that there are no guarantees with cancer, but there is hope. That doesn't stop them trying (very hard), every single day, to survive and be healthy, in mind, body and spirit.

For long-term survivors healing means wellness and they know they can both influence and affect that. With daily determination to stay well, they choose to live and

- o Meditate/do yoga/do Reiki
- o Drink organic vegetable juices
- o Eat fresh organic food
- o Exercise (even just walking)
- o Get enough rest
- o In as much as is possible, they live in the moment and stress free.

Long-term survivors believe that they will survive. Knowing that their thoughts affect their reality, they make a decision to do whatever it takes and whether consciously or sub-consciously, they decide to never give up. They focus all their energy on what is really important to them in life, what they can do and they let go of what they can't do. They hold on to the belief that everything is alright, in the same way that a drowning person clutches a life-line.

Long-term survivors work hard to keep their emotions balanced. They go within, confront and let go of blocked emotions like anger, past hurt, guilt, fear, lack of forgiveness and victimhood—knowing that not dealing with imbalanced emotions leads to illness. In other words, they deal with unresolved emotional issues. They learn to express their emotions—all of them.

Long-term survivors do many things that we should all be doing, even without the commitment to survival that they have. They rearrange their priorities. They accept the changes in their lives and are grateful for their lives, as they are and not as they wish they were. Within the framework in which they now find themselves, they re-invent themselves and embrace a new life. They count their blessings daily. They open their hearts and connect to the Universe. They believe that all is well in their world.

Long-term survivors are determined to live in the present, to live every day as if it were their last (the only day), to really enjoy life (in moderation), to be gentle with themselves, to treasure time, to relax, make time for activities that bring them joy, take time 'to be' and try to keep their lives balanced. They are intoxicated just with the joy and gift of being alive.

There are many things that long-term survivors no longer do. They no longer do anything that doesn't resonate with them, they no longer say 'yes' when they want to say 'no', they are non-fearful (most of the time!), they don't indulge in pessimism, don't think negative thoughts, don't hold on to the past, don't fight change, don't bury their feelings and emotions, don't sweat the small stuff, don't have room in their lives for complacency about their health, don't underestimate the self-healing abilities of their bodies, don't underestimate their own inner strength, don't think they are in control of their lives (it can take a while to internalize that one!) and they don't try to keep up anymore when they are not able to.

Long-term survivors are very motivated to make a difference in the world and they feel honoured to do their best to help other Champs on their journeys.

Long-term survivors understand that they need to take responsibility for their wellness, their health and their lives. They fully comprehend that every day is a choice. They have learned to slow down, flow with life and live one day at a time.

Most long-term survivors are grateful to have been given a second chance at life. They have goals and targets. They may desperately want to be around to raise their children, or to one day hold a grandchild in their arms, or to complete a career challenge, or to achieve a goal. Long-term survivors are usually pushed along life's path by a strong motivation and driving force to reach a destination or dream of one kind or another. This attitude appears to be vital.

Survival is hard work but people do survive, as a direct result of the skill of their medical team and an enormous effort on their own part. No one said that the road ahead would be easy, far from it, but it can be done. If you are reading this, and you are not a Champ, you may wonder if you could do this—well, the truth is, you could and would if your life depended on it, and how. For those of you who are already on the journey, you understand and fully accept that the journey doesn't end, you will be on it for the rest of your life. Life doesn't stretch on forever, as you may have once thought! Life will go on but we have learned that we don't know for how long. Long-term survival is about treasuring the gift of life (yours!) and choosing to spend the rest of your life living as opposed to dying.

I'M A SURVIVOR. I'M A LONG-TERM SURVIVOR . . .

HELP FROM 'THE OTHERS'!

Just imagine if Alexander Graham Bell could explain to you, personally, how the telephone works; or Steve Jobs took time to passionately share the visions that created his amazing Apple products; or Sarah Chang gave you a private concert and shared her techniques. Wouldn't it be mind-boggling and staggering to be in the company of these great minds and geniuses who mastered their 'trade' and know everything there is to know, and share, about their chosen field of expertise?

Here you are on the cancer journey, a little lost, majorly fearful of the unknown, floundering from minute to hour, test to scan, surgery to treatments and beyond. Help!

There are experts on hand to help you, free, with generous spirit, willing heart and at a moment's notice. Really! The true experts are, of course, the cancer survivors, the Champs who have already travelled the journey you are now on. Where in the world would you find more accurate accounts of what's involved, what to do, how one feels, where to find the most experienced healers and a measuring stick for your progress in mind, body and spirit?

The Champs who have done the journey before you and survived will fill this role and be a lot more than a walking 'google' on every aspect of what you are experiencing. It's like talking to someone who has just returned from the North Pole before setting off yourself.

The oncology nurse will prepare you for chemotherapy by telling you the expected side-effects of your particular drug cocktail, she'll inform you that you'll lose your hair, how many hours you'll be at the unit to receive your treatment and other important information.

A survivor on the other hand will fill in the gaps by pointing out that it's not just the hair on your head that will fall out but every hair on your body, including the hair in your nose, your eyebrows and eyelashes.

A survivor will tell you what things to bring with you, to the chemo unit, on the day of a treatment, which might help make being attached to a drip for ten to twelve hours, in a ward full of people who have cancer, a little more bearable.

A survivor will warn you that you'll most likely 'crash' when you come off steroids—every time. She'll talk you though finding veins 'in vain' every time you need to have a needle inserted into a possibly collapsed vein. She'll be the one to tell you to wear socks to theater for surgery as it's very cold in there. She'll advise you on little ideas to help you get through a thirty to forty minute session in a PET/CT tunnel, especially if you are slightly claustrophobic.

Your oncologist will ensure that your surgery is skillfully performed, that you are thoroughly checked out physically on a regular basis and that the best chemotherapy available to date will be used in making every effort to return you to full health.

But, you only see your oncologist once every three weeks for a brief visit. Who are you going to call on in the meantime?

- o Who will understand why you are falling apart emotionally?
- o Who will explain why, and not just advise you, to have your head shaved before your hair begins to fall out?
- o Who will know that jojoba oil soothes a red, sore and very irritated head from wearing a wig?
- o Who can direct you to a healer that will give you, the gift of gifts at this time, several hours free of pain and a soothed spirit thrown in for good measure?
- o Who will initiate you into the world of creating a strong, healthy body that is capable of staying strong through juicing, eating the right food, exercise, yoga, meditation and more?
- o Who can give you the name of the shops where you can buy colourful bandanas that completely and comfortably cover a bald head?
- o Who can ease you into an absurd upside-down world with such grace that you actually learn to live with cancer and carry on as normally as possible?

o Who will tell you that hot water will drive the pain in your 'Raynaud Syndrome' feet through the roof, so it's best to let go of relaxing, hot baths?

o Who will mention the word 'fear' at all, or listen and discuss yours so you can work your way around it and carry on?

o Who else really understands every single element, nuance, twist and turn of your current challenge and miraculously has solutions for almost every worry, problem and fear?

Even when a concrete solution is not to be found, the very fact that these women listen, understand, offer to help and are there any time you mail, text, call or reach out is more than enough to get you through the current 'dark' patch.

Cancer survivor women are a life-line. It's such a shame that doctors don't ask these very knowledgeable, experienced and treasure-troves of important and very useful information, to come and talk to Champs, who are starting, or are still doing the journey.

It's such a waste that survivor's insights are not collected by 'the team' (either oncologists, nurses, social workers or anyone who could put the insights to good use for others) when the women have finished their journeys. Every idea, observation and comment could enrich the protocol for helping the next Champs. Hopefully we all want to learn and improve the system so that others will have an easier 'ride' than we had, so that there will be less pain (emotional as well as physical) and more progress in the future.

I advise Champs who are just starting their journey to read survivor's stories, and through friends, or the internet, try to connect with survivors so they will have support and guidance as they travel their path. Every woman who has done the journey has learned, healed and grown. She has also seen for herself how the system, the journey and the benefits could be improved on, compared to what was available when she did her journey. Let's listen to and learn from these experts. Let not even one Champ's journey, effort and hardship have been in vain or be lost.

There isn't a day that goes by that I don't give thanks to (and for) the survivors who cushioned my journey, paved an easier way forward for me and were there for me, for whatever reason, 24/7, for as long as the cancer journey lasted and until my recovery was complete. Having seen up close, from my own personal encounter, how invaluable it was to have the torch of a survivor to light, support and explain the darkness of my path, it is now my turn to do the same for another woman, with love and gratitude that I'm here to do it.

HOW I CAN MAKE A
DIFFERENCE NOW . . .

BORN AGAIN

"Life is not about having the best of everything but about making the best of everything," Author unknown to me.

You died to your old life during the cancer journey. There is no going back—and would you really want to? The 'old' me could be casual and carefree about her health. The 'new' me is more joyful, relaxed, peaceful and stress-free. To have been given a second chance is an honour that I don't take lightly.

As I stood on the bridge that arched between my old life and my new, so much awareness and understanding flooded in. Now that the physical suffering was easing off, I realized that I was now at the point of learning readiness. It's as if, before, I was listening, whereas now I was listening, hearing and understanding too.

Cancer was a huge wake-up call for me. I'm awake and alert now and imagine I'll remain so for the rest of my life! I now know what's important. I'm careful about how I spend every moment of my very valuable time.

I know I have daily choices about whether I spend my time:

o Being joyful or fearful
o Being happy or miserable
o Being productive or lazy

o Being upbeat or negative
o Being active or passive
o Being grateful about feeling good or worrying about falling sick again
o Flowing with life or struggling to keep up
o Being part of healthy relationships or dysfunctional ones.

None of us has endless time, but I know I have today.

I may still look the same on the outside but inside I'm very different now. I don't think the same, feel the same or see things the same way. I know what I want and what I don't want (with a passion) and I want to live differently.

The cancer journey has enabled me to reinvent myself, so to speak. I have been given a golden opportunity to choose with whom I want to be (I stay away from negative, angry, judgmental, toxic people) and how I want to be in my life, in the world and with the people in my circle.

Before being born again I thought I was enjoying myself, but not every part of me was always fully in the fun of the moment, now it is. The new me knows how to enjoy herself fully. By this I mean being truly joyful in the moment of the joy. Life seems like so much more fun. I do what brings me joy. Inside I feel full of the joys of spring.

I know I must be the change I want to see in my life, therefore, I've changed at the most fundamental level of my being. My priorities have changed. There is no place in my life for being unnecessarily fearful, feeling guilty, people pleasing, acting like there is no choice, or doing anything that no longer 'fits' me. This does not mean that I've become selfish, no, I haven't. The change is that I'm in the centre of the picture, that is my own life, now. I'm so much more aware of the endless choices I have, all the time.

I feel that I've morphed into the person I feel I am inside and the person I was born to be. These days I measure the success of my life by:

o How well the relationships in my life are going
o The lessons I have learned and continue to learn
o The measure of love I give and can feel around me
o Whether my life is on track or not
o Whether I'm working towards what I was born to do or not.

You may not realize to what extent you have healed and grown till you wake up one morning and it hits you. Even if you continue to live within the same framework as you did pre-cancer, you will need to help your loved ones to see, understand and fully accept that things will never, ever be the same for you again.

Make sure you know the answers to the following questions:

1. Who am I now?
2. What do I want to stop doing?
3. What do I want to continue doing?

You need to be allowed to change, (it's safe to let go now) whatever the cost . . . even a relationship.

The only journey I do now is my own. Loving 'me' these days means putting my wellness before everything else.

I've grown accustomed to doing things more slowly, pacing myself, planning and executing my plans while I have energy (knowing that later I may not have), going out when I feel energetic and well enough to enjoy myself, taking naps, going to bed when I feel I need to, saying 'no', cancelling arrangements when I know I'm just not able, are all part of how I live my new life.

Having done the cancer journey, (learned, healed and grown), I now count my blessings, feel joyful and grateful with even more fervour. This is a new start for me, I've been born again. I am ready to plant the seeds, containing the endless, limitless possibilities of the entire forest of my future. A new 'me' has emerged, is evolving and will hopefully endure.

I'm now in the driver's seat of my life. I've offloaded great weights I'd been carrying around with me for the longest time.

I now enjoy the simple pleasures of life. Health, love, gratitude and peace define me. My heart smiles a lot more. I love more, understand more, accept more, enjoy more and forgive more readily. Life is too short not to.

Being in remission is a little like lying under a guillotine. There is the dread of recurrence. Days and days go by when cancer never crosses my mind but, naturally, I have moments of darkness when fear surges. I know that taking responsibility for my wellness is my best defense and the optimum I can do to keep myself healthy, well, able and strong. I invest lots of time, effort and energy in staying well. Once I feel I have left no stone unturned, I let go and flow with the certainty that I am not the one in control or in charge. Whatever will be, will be and in the meantime I want to get on with living and loving life to the full.

I'm a cancer survivor and I'm proud of it but I don't see or define myself as just that. Cancer is no longer the main focus of my day, my thoughts, my conversations or my life. I feel there is more to me than this one achievement. Surviving cancer is only part of my life, not all of it.

It's so important to me to make a difference in the world. I feel a huge need to help other Champs who follow my path on their cancer journey. That makes everything I endured worthwhile.

These days I feel strong and peaceful. I feel good most of the time and it's a joy. My life has, undoubtedly, changed for the better.

MY NEW LIFE . . .

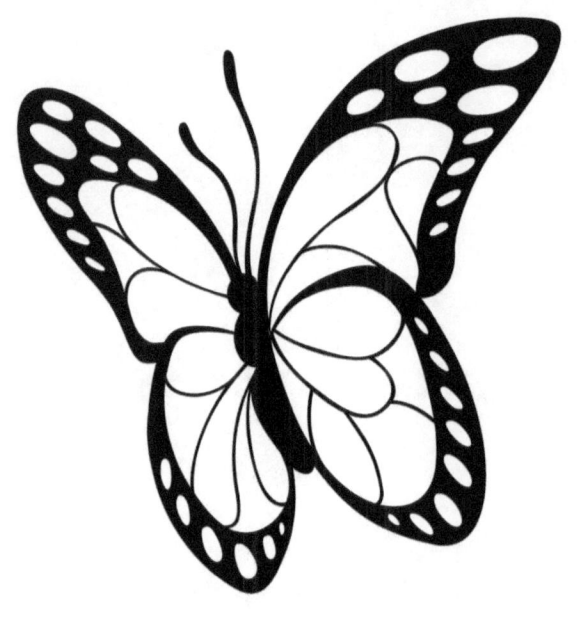

Even a butterfly spends time in the darkness of a cocoon before emerging triumphantly to freedom and light. In Mandarin Chinese, the butterfly symbolizes
LONG LIFE!

THE END . . .
WHICH, OF COURSE, IS ALSO A
NEW BEGINNING!

THANK YOU FOR THE GIFT OF YOUR PRECIOUS
TIME GIVEN TO READ *SLOW TRAIN*.
INFINITE LOVE, GRATITUDE & HEALTH TO YOU.

WHO AM I?

About the Author

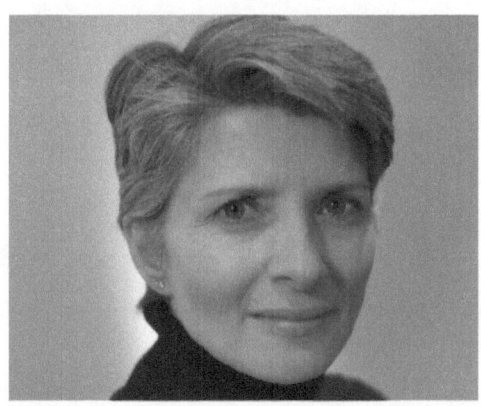

Dee Shemma is an ovarian cancer survivor. Prior to her cancer journey, she was an English teacher and writer.

Through the gift of cancer she has been re-born.

Dee currently lives, with her family, in Israel and can be reached at slowtrain6@gmail.com

POEMS-PRAYERS-PIECES

SCAN SCARED!

Tears overflow from my heart and down my
cheeks
As I call on all my loved ones, who have passed
away, by name.
Please come and hold me now in my time of
dread, terror, fear, anxiety, worry and panic.
Do you know any well-connected angels yet?
Not knowing what's going on inside me is too
much for me now.
Facing another PET/CT doesn't fit.
I've finally figured out what life is all about,
How the Universe works,
Uncovered who I am,
Discovered what I was born to do,
Learned so many lessons,
Realized I can make a difference,
And untangled so much wisdom.
I'm ready at last so don't steal away my time
Don't snatch my chance to live.
Please, I so humbly beg—bestow on me the
treasured time I so soulfully seek.
If all else fails
No matter what the results reveal
Grant me the grace to graciously greet my news
with gratitude,

Acceptance and peace.
I'm not just asking or praying, it's more than
even haggling—
I'm begging and pleading, with the greatest
humility.

Dee

OVERCOME!

May you be swathed in love
May you be protected and healed
Trust that all is as it's meant to be
Be assured that you are exactly in the right place
at the right time
Breathe in health, serenity, tranquility and peace
Exhale anything that for you, today, is toxic
Feel and bathe in the love that surrounds you
Give gratitude for all your endless gifts
Relax, laugh, enjoy and have fun!

Dee

HELP ME!

I ask you to help me to accept what is happening
to me.
Help me to be strong when I feel fearful and
tired.
Help me to get out of bed and stay out for as
long as I can.
Help me to think positive thoughts.
Help me to see things differently:
Sick → challenged
Tired → need to rest
Afraid → all is well.

Dee

LOVE THE LESSON!

Knowing that I make my own reality,
Help my light to shine brighter than ever at this
time,
So that my learning may be a catalyst for change
in the lives of others,
Help me to remember that I chose this
challenge long before I was born,
That it is part of my journey, my soul's
evolvement.
It's just another lesson.
I embrace it with gratitude.

Dee

AFFIRMATIONS

The affirmations that I said on my journey:

o "My body is healthy, well, able and strong. The surgeries, chemotherapy and alternative treatments are healing my body to perfect, vibrant and lasting health."

o "My name is Dee and today I choose to balance my CA125 (ovarian cancer marker) level. My body is a perfect healing organism and so it is."

o "The nerve endings in my hands and feet are in perfect working order."

o "I am healthy, happy and healed."

o "I am a cancer survivor."

o "My body is a perfect healing organism."

Make up your own affirmations in accordance with your needs, just remember to:

o Keep them short
o In the present tense
o Refer to your goal
o Avoid the use of negatives

o   They must be only about you and your needs
o   Be specific
o   Say them as many times as possible every day.

THE 'FAMOUS FOLDER'

Life will be a lot less complicated and easier to manage, if you start your journey with a 'famous folder' (maybe you call it a ring-binder in your country)!

It's easier to organize it early on the journey, when you have only a few pages to sort. Choose a colour for the folder that is pleasing to you, light and cheery. I decorated mine with a smiley and a spiral because of what they symbolized to me, they were reminders.

Here are a few tips on how to make the 'famous folder' more manageable and user friendly:

o Place about forty poly-pocket plastic page protectors in the folder
o Organize all the medical pages, reports, results and information in chronological order
o Place each page in a separate pocket, unless a few of the pages relate to the same test or report, in which case, they should be placed in the same pocket
o I generally keep the conventional medicine pages at the front of the folder and all the alternative medicine pages at the back, just for easy access to them in a hurry
o I keep a page at the back of the folder for useful phone numbers:

- ✓ Immediate family members
- ✓ Family doctor
- ✓ Gynecologist
- ✓ Gyne/oncologist
- ✓ Surgeon
- ✓ Blood Test Centre
- ✓ Gyne/oncology unit
- ✓ Chemotherapy unit
- ✓ Healers
- ✓ Pharmacy
- ✓ Health Insurance/Health Care Provider
- ✓ Any other number that, for you, is significant

o Place the notebook that you bring to doctor's visits in one of the pockets

o On a separate page, entitled PROGRESS PICTURE, you can write the following headings:
  - ✓ The date
  - ✓ CA125 level (or the marker name for your type of cancer)
  - ✓ Marker level up or down (compared to last blood test result)
  - ✓ Thank you (under which you will write your desired marker level)

  This way you can monitor your progress at a glance

o It's a great idea to keep a page just as a calendar of events. I know this is a great idea simply because I **didn't** do it! Every new doctor, specialist, consultant, surgeon, and medical 'helper' of every kind that you meet, for the first time, will ask you to fill him in on the 'story' of your illness. They don't need your life story, just dates, so this page can save a lot of time. All you need to list are the dates of the most significant stations:

- ✓ Your original diagnosis
- ✓ Any biopsies or surgeries
- ✓ When chemotherapy started
- ✓ When chemotherapy ended
- ✓ CT, PET/CT or MRI scans
- ✓ Any other major events that you feel are significant.

I won't tell you when you'll need to bring your folder with you because you'll need it **every** time you go anywhere that's even remotely connected, in any way, with your wellness, healing, health and cancer journey. I only once left mine at home and yes, you guessed already, that was the very day I was asked for so many details, reports and information! Never again, I promised myself, would the 'famous folder' get to stay home alone!

CHEMOTHERAPY CHECKLIST

It was an important comfort to pack all the right things for the full day at the hospital (8 a.m. till about 6 p.m.). I normally packed:

- o A book
- o A journal/notebook and pen
- o My iPod, with podcasts, music and meditation at the ready
- o Photographs of loved ones
- o Cards that had been sent to me with wonderful energy
- o My favourite aromatherapy oil. Sometimes there can be a smell that's unpleasant, for you, or no smell at all and you can adjust your environment to something pleasing, restful and reminiscent of home with your oils
- o All relevant medical papers. I highly recommend just bringing your 'famous folder' with all your medical history (for this illness) to date in it
- o Your phone. You will send and receive messages and calls from loved ones throughout the very long day
- o Some money, there will be a cafeteria
- o Sanitizer, wipes, tissues
- o A bag that can be used for rubbish
- o Food for the day. Food is served at the hospital but if you have preferences, or

are following a special healthy diet, then bring your own. I normally brought soup, a wholegrain sandwich, vegetable sticks, fruit, dried fruit, a salad, lots of water and tea
- o I always brought two china mugs, one for me and one for any friend that might visit!
- o Consider the following before choosing what to wear:

  - ✓ You'll be wearing what you choose for the entire day, whether you are sitting or lying down. I once made the mistake of wearing a sweat-shirt with a hood, which was so uncomfortable later when I was lying down and trying to sleep
  - ✓ I suggest a layered look. If you wear a cardigan or sweatshirt over a t-shirt, remember that the sleeves of the sweatshirt need to be loose enough to slip easily over your IV needle, if you feel too hot or cold. The IV needle could be positioned anywhere from your elbow to your knuckles!
  - ✓ I found pashminas to be very useful in that they could be easily thrown over my shoulders, my feet, my pillow or wherever required
  - ✓ I feel that loose, comfortable elastic-waisted 'bottoms' are best. Think about it, you'll be either sitting or lying all day. You'll have to take the IV stand with you

to the bathroom and eat with it too, so in theory, you'll only have full use of one hand for the duration, therefore, struggling with zips and buttons may present a challenge

✓ I found slip-on shoes, like clogs, crocs or flip-flops to be easiest to manage, on the many trips from bed to bathroom; remembering again that lacing or buckling a shoe would not have been easy with one hand

✓ I always wore socks as the air-con can get cold as the day wears on, in an enclosed room.

o Needless to add, like everything else in life, you learn as you go along and having made mistakes with what I brought and didn't bring to the unit with me, with how I packed my bags and where I placed my gear for the day, I got it right in the end. I learned that it was important to pack the food in one bag, items I'd like to have immediate and continuous access to in a second bag and the rest of the stuff in a third bag.

Good luck! Let today be about you. Be gentle with yourself. You are not alone. For today, just 'be'. Sending love and light to you, dear Champ.